MW00616507

HOW
TO
HAVE
A BABY

The essential unbiased guide
to pregnancy, birth and beyond

HOW
TO
HAVE
A BABY

DR SARA KAYAT

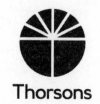

Thorsons

Thorsons
An imprint of HarperCollins*Publishers*
1 London Bridge Street
London SE1 9GF

www.harpercollins.co.uk

HarperCollins*Publishers*
Macken House, 39/40 Mayor Street Upper
Dublin 1, D01 C9W8, Ireland

First published by Thorsons 2024

1 3 5 7 9 10 8 6 4 2

© Dr Sara Kayat 2024
Illustrations by Liane Payne

Dr Sara Kayat asserts the moral right to be identified as the author of this work
A catalogue record of this book is available from the British Library

ISBN 978-0-00-862716-4

Printed and bound in the UK using 100%
renewable electricity at CPI Group (UK) Ltd

All rights reserved. No part of this publication may be reproduced, stored
in a retrieval system, or transmitted, in any form or by any means, electronic,
mechanical, photocopying, recording or otherwise, without the
prior written permission of the publishers.

While the author of this work has made every effort to ensure that the information
contained in this book is as accurate and up-to-date as possible at the time of
publication, medical and pharmaceutical knowledge is constantly changing and the
application of it to particular circumstances depends on many factors. Therefore, it is
recommended that readers always consult a qualified medical specialist for individual
advice. This book should not be used as an alternative to seeking specialist medical
advice which should be sought before any action is taken. The author and publishers
cannot be held responsible for any errors and omissions that may be found in the text,
or any actions that may be taken by a reader as a result of any reliance on the
information contained in the text which is taken entirely at the reader's own risk.

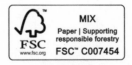

This book is produced from independently certified FSC™ paper
to ensure responsible forest management.

For more information visit: www.harpercollins.co.uk/green

CONTENTS

Introduction 1

Chapter 1: Pre-pregnancy 4

Chapter 2: Early Pregnancy 14

Chapter 3: Pregnancy 29

Chapter 4: Preparing for Labour 64

Chapter 5: Labour 87

Chapter 6: Postnatal, Baby and You 128

Chapter 7: Feeding your Baby 182

Chapter 8: Sleep 229

Chapter 9: Weaning 251

Chapter 10: Teething 268

Chapter 11: Baby Vaccinations 274

Chapter 12: Milestones 280

Final Word 287

Endnotes 289

Acknowledgements 306

Index 307

INTRODUCTION

Welcome to an insight into my mini family. I am a doctor who qualified in 2009 and became a GP five years later. I'd always thought general practice was about verrucas, ear wax and roll-neck jumpers, but during a medical school rotation I was placed under the care of a brilliant GP who showed me the heart, soul, necessity and complexity of this specialty. As well as being a great doctor, though, she also had a life. She had photos of her family all around her room, she had trinkets from her travels and interesting books on her shelf. She inspired me to become a GP, but she also reminded me that I could succeed academically and still have a family that I could spend time with and adore. So now, over a decade after that rotation, I sit here writing this book, as a happy NHS and private GP, resident doctor on *This Morning*, wife to a never-ageing (seriously, he still looks like he's 20!) goofball Rupert, cat owner to Mlem and, most importantly of all, mother to my absolute legend of a three-year-old boy, Harris.

I remember very distinctly the day I found out I was pregnant. We had been 'trying' for a few months so it wasn't exactly a shock, but it still took me quite unawares. My husband and I were driving to the in-laws' house to celebrate a family member being discharged from the cancer ward at hospital that day, and I had just received a text message from the Mother-in-Law saying, 'can't wait to see you both, champagne is chilling'. Imagining the cork popping off, a bell rang in the distant ether of my brain as I remembered my period was due some time that week. I had been feeling a little rank the two days prior and just couldn't sleep, but despite being a GP I hadn't really put two and two together.

As we were driving, I asked my husband to pull over at a Tesco so I could buy a pregnancy test, as I really bloody wanted that champagne and I wasn't going to let an imagined pregnancy stand in the way! I picked up the absolute cheapest of cheap pregnancy tests (think Soviet War rationing-type device), assuming that if they're good enough for the NHS, they're good enough for me, and I made my way to the scuzziest of supermarket toilets. This is the kind of test that you need a pot to pee into, then you need to pipette said urine onto it, rather than the much easier (and more expensive) pee-on-the-stick types, but optimistically I reckoned that with my coordination, pelvic floor strength and flexibility, I could make it work.

Suffice to say, the scuzzy toilet was significantly damper after my attempt, and I was none the wiser. But it was ok, though, because for the princely sum of £1.99 they gave me two pregnancy tests in the kit. So I thought, I'll just wait till I get to the in-laws' house and do it again in a more controlled and hygienic environment. We arrived to a champagne reception, and I had to pretend that I was SO very desperate to pee that I simply could not hold it for long enough to have a 'cheers' and a sip, and I escaped to the toilet. There I performed the 'experiment' with a lot more dignity and precision, but I couldn't tell if there were two lines on the test, with one being exceptionally faint, or if it was just one line and the second line was in my hopeful imagination. I left the test hidden behind a cabinet in the bathroom and asked my husband to go in and have a look at it and tell me what he thought. He came back out of the toilet looking flushed and entirely perplexed, like I had asked him to work out a quadratic equation. He didn't know either. The remainder of the day was spent accidentally spilling a lot of champagne (what a waste) and 'mistakenly' swapping my glass with my husband's. At one point I even blamed the neighbour's children, who had also come over to join in the festivities, for knocking a glass out of my hand. Yes, this was a new low.

On the way home, I stopped off at the same Tesco and forked out a ridiculous £11 for a 'proper' test, and on arriving home I did the deed and the word POSITIVE sprung up (thank the Lord I didn't have to interpret any cryptic faint lines). I opened up my laptop, self-referred to the antenatal hospital in which I was born and ordered my Transport for London 'baby on board' badge.

Everything was about to change. Despite being a self-professed Mother Nature type who is often quoted as saying 'I was born to be a mum', as well as having the title of doctor under my belt – who has helped lots of mothers through their pre- and postnatal journeys – I was entirely unprepared.

No amount of time spent on YouTube watching births, episodes of *Motherland*, or sitting in cold church halls for antenatal classes will brace you for the enormity of what that extra line on the pregnancy test means for your life. My aim in writing this book is that by sharing my own honest experiences, with a hefty medical slant, you will hopefully feel more confident about the bits you can control, have a better understanding of the science behind all the variables so you can make more informed decisions, get a few practical tips, have a laugh, and ultimately realise that even doctors are as scared as you are when pregnancy happens to them. We are all in this together, holding each other's clammy, anxious hands!

CHAPTER 1

PRE-PREGNANCY BE PREPARED

I knew when it was time for us to start trying to conceive. We had been married for two years, together for six, and we were in a good place. Work was stable, we lived somewhere that could accommodate a little one, we were healthy and, importantly, we were happy. I thought this was a lovely environment to bring a child into. I came off contraception, but I didn't fall pregnant straight away.

As a GP, I regularly sit with an anxious woman of childbearing age who has been trying to conceive for the last three months with no success, and almost verbatim I let the words 'in those having regular sex, 84 per cent will fall pregnant within a year'[1] roll off my tongue. This is meant to reassure a woman that three months is not that long, and they should come back in a year if it still hasn't happened so we can then investigate the cause. I had never appreciated how long a year is when you've finally made the decision that *now* is when you want a baby. I didn't want to wait, so I decided to take investigations into my own hands and started wearing a device that measured my skin temperature, resting pulse, breathing rate, heart rate variability ratio and my sleep. All these parameters change depending on where you are in your cycle.

In order to fall pregnant you need to have sex in the days leading up to and including ovulation (when your egg is released). Sperm can survive within your female tracts for up to a week, so having sex at any time in the week prior may mean you fall pregnant, but your chances are at their highest on the day before and day of ovulation. The books all say we ovulate on day 14 of our cycle, so the world rampantly has sex around this magical day and expects miracles, but this doesn't take into account the fact that we are all different. Armed with all of the information from my device, I was able to see that I wasn't ovulating on day 14 at all, but actually on day 18, so there was a lot of ineffective (albeit lovely) intercourse being had!

I know lots of people dislike the medicalisation of the baby-making process and prefer to keep it impromptu and romantic, but honestly, I really enjoyed getting to know and understand my body on a whole new level. I went from thinking that a period was a total pain in the arse to actually something empowering, because in really coming to terms with my cycle and knowing when I was having hormonal surges or dips helped me to plan my weeks – from the type of exercise I should do, to knowing when my hormonal waves would make me feel more confident in myself so I could try to book in important discussions with the boss, or when I would be more emotional and want to be around supportive friends. Within three months of wearing this device, I was pregnant – though I hasten to add that it's impossible to say conclusively whether this was because of the information I was getting from it or that it would have happened at this point anyway.

Being in the position of actively trying to fall pregnant, I was able to prepare myself for pregnancy. Women who are healthier at conception have a better chance of becoming pregnant, having a safe and healthy pregnancy, and giving birth to a blooming baby. To ensure optimum preconception health, there are a number of factors I would advise being aware of:

1. Start taking folic acid *before* you become pregnant

Folic acid is a manmade form of folate, a B vitamin that occurs naturally in foods like Brussels sprouts, broccoli, yeast extract, spinach, black eye peas and chickpeas. It helps to protect against neural tube defects (NTDs) in your baby, where the spine of the foetus does not develop properly in the womb. The most common example of this is spina bifida, where one or more of the bones in the spine fail to develop fully, leaving gaps in the spine and damaging the nerves and cord. This can mean that the baby suffers with paralysis, and it can affect their bladder and bowel control too. However, we know that women who take 400mcg of folic acid during early pregnancy are much less likely to have babies with NTD[2] (if you have a Body Mass Index (BMI) – see below – of 30 or over you will need to take 5mg). As such, it is recommended that you start taking folic acid before you fall pregnant, ideally two to three months before, so that you build up your levels of folic acid to a level that protects your baby, up until 12 weeks of pregnancy.

2. Try to get to a healthy weight

Being a healthy weight in pregnancy is important because being either over- or underweight can affect your fertility, increase your risks of problems during pregnancy and pose risks to your baby. Using your height and weight we can work out your BMI, which is a rudimentary way to determine if you are a healthy weight. BMI can be a flawed measurement, as it doesn't take into account the fact that muscle is denser than fat – weighing about 18 per cent more – so I recommend an individualised approach. BMI alone, without measuring other health determinants, might also not be a particularly useful screening tool. A study by Oxford University[3] showed that the increased risks in pregnancy associated with obesity were actually fairly modest in women who did not have other conditions like high blood pressure or diabetes, or who had had previous Caesarean sections. The risks were even lower if the woman had given birth before. Therefore, the risks are not the same for all women in the same BMI bracket.

Additionally, your BMI should not be used as a tool for humiliation. Yes, we need to be informed of the possible effects that being over- or underweight can have on our reproductive journeys, but during an already vulnerable time, sensitivity is required in communicating this. Furthermore, if you have any underlying conditions that affect your weight, it may be that you have no control over it, and the weight 'guilt trip' may feel even more unfair.

There is, rightly, the expectation that as healthcare professionals we should discuss the risks of a high or low BMI with pregnant women and give dietary and exercise advice as per the National Institute for Health and Care Excellence (NICE) guidelines. However, the way we communicate risk in pregnancy is important, because the psychological impact of our words can also be influential to our wellbeing. Whilst it is my duty to provide the information as below, I don't want you to come away from this chapter feeling stigmatised. If you are struggling with your weight, or you would like to discuss the potential impact of your weight on pregnancy further, you should talk to your midwife about this.

Overweight:
- Having a BMI of 25 and over can reduce your risk of falling pregnant. This is because overweight or obese women produce more of a hormone called leptin, which can affect the regulation of the sex hormones androgen and oestrogen, and in turn it increases the risk of irregular menstrual cycles and not ovulating.
- During pregnancy an elevated BMI can increase your risk of health conditions like pre-eclampsia. Having a BMI of 35 or over doubles your risk of this condition compared to a woman with a BMI of below 25. Being overweight also increases your risk of other conditions, such as gestational diabetes, blood clots, requiring an emergency Caesarean section and heavier bleeding after birth. However, it is not recommended to limit your intake of food groups and go on a significant diet during pregnancy, which is why it is best to do this *before* falling pregnant.
- A high BMI can affect the way your baby develops, increasing the risk of miscarriage, a stillbirth or premature birth and having a baby with a high birth weight, which can be carried on into adulthood.

Underweight:
- Having a BMI of under 18.5 can also reduce your chance of falling pregnant, due to hormonal imbalances, whereby you produce lower levels of oestrogen, affecting your cycle and whether you ovulate regularly or at all.
- It can also affect your pregnancy, resulting in an increased risk of miscarriage.
- Babies can be born premature, have a low birth weight and have an increased risk of the condition gastroschisis, where the stomach doesn't develop properly.

3. Learn your family history

My husband and I often discussed whether our baby would have his blue eyes or my dark complexion, or perhaps my weird ET toes, but really, at the top of the discussion list for familial traits should have been whether either of us had any family history of birth defects, developmental disabilities or genetic conditions. That may not be as simple as saying we have no obvious conditions, but rather delving a few generations back, if you are able to, to see if you might be a carrier of a condition.

In human beings our sex cells (our sperm and eggs) are known as gametes, and each gamete carries 23 chromosomes, which on fusing completes our 46 chromosomes. So this means that you have two copies of every gene – one from your mother and one from your father. This is excellent, because if one copy is broken due to a certain condition, you still have the other. So whilst you still carry this broken gene and are called a 'carrier' of a condition, you do not actually suffer with the condition itself due to the other healthy copy. However, carriers are still able to pass that broken gene down to their offspring, and this is how some conditions are unknowingly passed down to the next generation.

Let's say Mum carries a broken gene; she has a 50 per cent chance of that gene being passed down to her baby. Even if the baby is in that unlucky 50 per cent, it isn't usually much of a problem as you are likely to still get a healthy copy of that gene from Dad, so your baby ends up just being a carrier. However, if Dad also has this broken gene, there is a 50 per cent chance that he too will pass it to his baby. This means there is a 25 per cent chance that the broken gene will be passed down to the baby from both Mum and Dad, resulting in a baby who suffers with the disease. That's a pretty high risk when you take into consideration how serious the conditions can be – for example, cystic fibrosis or sickle cell anaemia.

Essentially, we all have a number of broken genes, and if you are unlucky enough to mate with someone who happens to have this same break, then the baby is at risk. Genetics isn't always as simple as this, and there are different ways in which traits and diseases can be passed down, but this gives the simplest example of why we should try to be aware of our family medical histories and ask the questions wherever we are able to.

4. Review your medications

There are some medications you might be taking that may affect your chances of falling pregnant, and others that may affect your baby once pregnant.

The medicines that affect fertility can do so through different modalities – dysregulating your cycle, stopping ovulation and affecting your egg reserve. Commonly prescribed medications that can affect fertility include some antidepressants, antiepileptics and steroids. But it is not just about the prescribed medications, others, such as non-steroidal anti-inflammatory drugs (NSAIDs), which are commonly purchased as over-the-counter medications and include the frequently used ibuprofen, may affect fertility. Studies have found that the long-term or high-dose use of ibuprofen can disrupt the menstrual cycle and therefore affect fertility[4].

Many women also undergo acupuncture and use Chinese medicine to help increase their chances of falling pregnant. Some studies support the use of Chinese medicine in fertility[5], though there is little evidence that acupuncture will increase the likelihood of conception[6]. Whilst there is no harm to patients receiving acupuncture, there does seem to be some concern around herbal medicines[7]. St John's wort, echinacea and ginkgo biloba are some herbs that may negatively affect your chances of conceiving[8].

This one might sound obvious, but stop your contraception! Although we spend all of our twenties and thirties terrified that if we miss one single pill we are instantly going to fall pregnant (and this can, of course, be true for some!), for many of us, it can take around three months for the natural cycle to return. Whilst you do not have to wait these three months to attempt to conceive, it is often recommended that you wait for one period before trying to get pregnant. This is not the withdrawal bleed that you will have straight after stopping, but the first natural cycle. If you do fall pregnant before this, don't worry, it is very unlikely that there would be any harm to your baby, it may just make it a little more difficult for the doctor to estimate how many weeks' pregnant you are. It is worth knowing that whilst fertility can return instantly after stopping/removing most contraception, it can take a little longer with the contraception injection, so factor this into your plans.

Once pregnant, most medicines that are taken do cross the placenta, reaching the baby, so it is important to review the medications you're on before you fall pregnant, to ensure none of them can affect your little one. It may be tempting to just stop all medicines once you've found out you're pregnant, but it is very important that you don't do this without speaking to your doctor first. Whilst we generally want our pregnant patients to be on as few medications as possible, it is worth knowing that the majority of women in the developed world use at least one medication during pregnancy[9]. The discussion you have with your doctor should include weighing up the risks and benefits of your medication, about the safety of each, and whether you can swap this to something safer or, even better, try non-pharmaceutical approaches. This is the case for both physical and mental health conditions.

5. Stop the boozing

I can't really preach about this, I was in Croatia celebrating my husband's 40th birthday when we conceived Harris, and there was alcohol involved. From the day I found out, however, until the day I popped, a drop didn't pass my lips – in part to try to annul the guilt I had for the conception drinking sesh, but also because the thought of drinking just made me feel nauseous.

The NHS advises you to not drink alcohol at all if you are pregnant or trying to conceive, and in an ideal world this is what we would all adhere to. However, given that the majority of the drinking population is of reproductive age, it is not uncommon for those trying to conceive to regularly consume alcohol. It is easy to tut at this, but, as discussed, it can take up to a year or more in some cases to fall pregnant, and for many women this duration of sobriety can feel isolating. It can also be very difficult to conceal your reasons for being tee-total if you don't want to let everyone know that you're trying for a baby. This probably explains why a study of over 5,000 pregnant women found that those with an intended pregnancy were only 31 per cent less likely to consume alcohol in pregnancy than those with unintended pregnancies[10].

The question is, why can't you drink alcohol? Again, the answer lies in how it might affect your fertility and then how it might affect your unborn baby.

The effects of alcohol on fertility have been poorly researched, but studies in humans and animals have found changes to ovulation, ovarian reserve and the menstrual cycle with chronic alcohol intake[11]. It is likely due to the fact that alcohol increases the reproductive hormones oestradiol, testosterone and luteinizing hormone, with greater increases seen in women who binge-drink.

However, despite these noted changes, multiple studies have actually found no relationship between moderate alcohol consumption and fertility[12]. There have been some smaller studies which do suggest a decreased chance of achieving a clinical pregnancy in those that drink some alcohol versus no alcohol[13], but larger, more robust studies have found no significant consistencies.

To play devil's advocate, a retrospective study[14] of almost 40,000 pregnant women actually reported a shortened time to pregnancy in women who consumed a moderate amount of alcohol compared with those who did not drink at all! This may be due to the 'relaxation card'. I have seen numerous patients, living stressful and difficult lives, who have consulted with me, struggling to conceive. They've done everything by the book – stopped drinking, maintained a healthy lifestyle, worked out their fertile windows, taken all the supplements – but somewhere along the line they have understandably become significantly stressed by the whole process. The relationship between stress and infertility is well documented[15], though it is less understood whether there is a direct causal link between stress and infertility, and the research is conflicting. However, it's a great opportunity to really look after yourself, taking this time to use that spa voucher you were given for your birthday last year and have yet to enjoy, book into a Yin yoga class, or send your partner out on an errand and enjoy a bit of quiet and time alone on the sofa. Self-care isn't just a popular cliche to bandy around, it truly is important.

Whilst there might be a grey area around drinking and fertility, the negative effects of alcohol on the foetus are better understood. Alcohol readily passes across the placenta to the amniotic fluid and foetus, but the foetus will actually be exposed to higher concentrations of alcohol than the mother. This is because the foetus metabolises the alcohol more slowly, so it accumulates in the amniotic fluid. Studies have shown that mothers who drink more than one to two units of alcohol a day during pregnancy have babies with a greater risk of preterm birth, low birth weight and being small for gestational age[16]. The other risk associated with chronic alcohol consumption and pregnancy is foetal alcohol syndrome (FAS). This term describes a group of symptoms that can occur in a baby who was exposed to alcohol prenatally and whose brain development was affected. The problems with their neurological development can result in learning difficulties, movement and balance problems, hyperactivity and attention deficit, as well as hearing and vision problems. They also suffer from abnormal growth, often being smaller at birth and shorter than the average adult, have characteristic facial features including a head that is smaller than average, small eyes, a thin upper lip and a smooth area between the nose and upper lip.

We do not know what the safe amount is that you can drink, only that the more you drink the greater the risk. FAS is entirely preventable by avoiding alcohol during pregnancy and, as such, the safest approach is not to drink alcohol at all whilst trying to conceive or when you are pregnant.

But what if you hadn't planned on falling pregnant?

Not everyone is as much of a control freak as me, and in England 45 per cent of pregnancies are unplanned (or associated with feelings of ambivalence)[17]. So, if this is you, that's ok, you haven't doomed your baby! Just start taking folic acid as soon as you find out, stop boozing, don't try to suddenly lose weight, and book an appointment with your GP as soon as possible to discuss any medications. If you are concerned about any developmental or genetic family history, your doctor will be able to review this with you and refer you to a geneticist, if appropriate.

PRE-PREGNANCY: A TIRED MAMMA'S SUMMARY

Folic acid: start taking folic acid supplements before conception to prevent neural tube defects in the baby. Ideally, begin 2 to 3 months before conception and continue to take it until the twelfth week of pregnancy.

Healthy weight: maintaining a healthy weight is important for both partners, as being either overweight or underweight has an impact on fertility and pregnancy outcomes.

Family medical history: having as much knowledge as possible about your and your partner's family medical history is essential to identify potential genetic conditions or birth defects that may be passed down to the baby, how genetic traits are inherited, and the importance of being aware of carrier status.

Medications: it is important to review any medications you are taking, including over-the-counter drugs and herbal supplements, that could affect your fertility or the baby's development. Discuss these with a healthcare provider before conception.

Alcohol: while the effects of moderate alcohol consumption on fertility are debated, the risks to the foetus are well-documented, including low birth weight, preterm birth and foetal alcohol syndrome.

CHAPTER 2

EARLY PREGNANCY BE PREPARED

Now onto the <insert as appropriate> fun/terrifying/nauseating/ exhilarating part! You are pregnant. What the hell do you do now?!

Firstly, celebrate. Everyone's journey to get here is different – it may have been a breeze, or you might have been trying to conceive for a long time – but the end point is the same: you are pregnant. Take in the moment, breathe, hug, take photos of the pregnancy test and the non-existent bump. Then it's on to the practicalities …

CHOOSING YOUR HOSPITAL

The next step in your antenatal journey is to decide which maternity unit you would like to register your pregnancy with. In the UK you can generally give birth in either a labour ward, a birth centre or at home. But whichever you choose for your birth plan, on the NHS you still need a referral to a hospital to begin your antenatal assessments and scans. This is usually done by self-referral, by going onto your chosen hospital's website and filling out a simple form. If this is at all difficult, or your hospital doesn't have this facility, your GP can do the referral for you. A GP referral may also be more appropriate if you have any complicated medical or social issues that you think would be best explained to the hospital team by a healthcare professional.

Choosing the hospital can seem daunting, especially if you live in a big city where there are several to choose from. However, if you live in an area where hospitals are spread out and you don't want to travel long distances, your options may be more limited. You are free to choose any maternity service, so do not feel obliged to pick your most local provider if you have reservations about it.

I decided to choose the hospital that I was born in. There were a few reasons for this. First and foremost, it has an excellent maternity unit – I knew a couple of gynaecologists who worked there and they highly recommended it. Secondly, it was fairly close, perhaps not the closest, but near enough that I could get there within 30 minutes, if needed. Thirdly, a sentimental and emotional side. My mother hasn't been well for a while, so she hasn't been able to be part of my pregnancy or motherhood in the way I would have loved her to be. I wanted to do something that made me feel closer to her, and I thought that perhaps walking down the same corridors as she did, lying down for my ultrasounds in the same rooms as she did, and eventually giving birth in the same ward as she did would give me some of the comfort I needed.

What works for you?

You may have other priorities in choosing the right maternity hospital for you, which might include:

- Does the hospital have a birthing centre as well as a labour ward/ birthing pool/birthing chair?
- Will there be any restrictions? Such as the number of birthing partners, is your partner allowed to stay overnight, what's the visitors' policy?
- What pain relief is available?
- Does the hospital have a special baby unit or would the baby need to be transferred somewhere if there was a problem?

Your GP might be able to answer some of these questions, or at least discuss feedback they have had from other patients. Peer knowledge is also very useful, so speak to your friends who have had babies at the different hospitals. They will be able to offer first-hand insight into their experiences, though, of course, remember that everyone's pregnancies and labour are different and what happened to them may not necessarily happen to you.

But here's the important part – you are not tied into anything, you can always register with a hospital and then, if you aren't happy with the service or you're not getting positive vibes, you can swap. Your midwife or GP will be able to help coordinate that for you.

THE BOOKING VISIT

Now that you've booked in with a maternity service, providing you are feeling well, there's nothing else you need to do unprompted, so sit back and try to embrace the journey.

You will receive your first appointment with the midwife, which is usually termed your booking visit or appointment. Most people will have their first appointment by the time they're 10 weeks pregnant. However, if you have underlying health conditions, such as diabetes, you may be seen more quickly. If you only found out you're pregnant after this 10-week mark, contact your GP as soon as possible so they can help to expedite an appointment.

Where you have the appointment can depend on your local area; sometimes it is at the hospital, GP surgery, children's centre or your home. For me it was at a children's centre, which are these magical places I never knew existed until my pregnancy, despite having lived opposite one for five years – I thought it was just some weird portacabin in the park! They are places where local families with young children can go to enjoy the facilities and receive any support they need. It was so good to know about their existence, as Harris and I continue to go regularly. We get to hang out with other kids and parents, use their toys, attend music classes and I get little tips about parenting – from teeth brushing to effective reading – and this is all for free!

This first midwife appointment is an important one, as it gives you the chance to highlight any concerns you have about your pregnancy so the team can ensure you get the right support. The questions they will ask at first seem fairly straightforward; such as where you live, your support network, your relationship with the baby's father, your job, your health, as well as your smoking, drug and alcohol use. They will discuss the antenatal care you will receive, classes you can go to and exercises – including pelvic floor, diet, breastfeeding, options of where to have your baby and the benefits you're entitled to when pregnant.

They will also need to go into more sensitive matters, including any history of domestic abuse, mental health concerns and history of Female Genital Mutilation (FGM). These can feel like very difficult things to open up about to someone you don't know. I often suggest to my patients that if there is a topic that they know they will clam up about but is important to discuss, they should write it all down before. They can then either read from it themselves, which can help to remove the pressure, or just hand it to the midwife to read.

This appointment is also an opportunity to do some examinations.

You will have your height and weight measured to work out your BMI. As discussed on page 6, your BMI can be a risk factor for complications to both mother and baby, so you may be offered more frequent tests, including for gestational diabetes, blood pressure monitoring and ultrasound scans. You should also be offered support to try to limit weight gain, though weight loss and dieting during pregnancy is not advised.

You will also have your blood pressure checked; this is because of a condition called pre-eclampsia. This can affect pregnant women usually from the second half of their pregnancy, resulting in high blood pressure and protein in your urine. Most cases are mild and easily treated, but if it is not caught early it can lead to complications for mum and baby, including eclampsia, which are fits. This condition is rare but it can be life-threatening.

You will have a blood test. This will be to test for three infections: HIV, hepatitis B and syphilis. These are infections that can be passed on to your baby, so we test it early in case we need to start treatment and limit that risk. You may have other tests to ensure you are not anaemic, and you will also be offered a blood test to check your blood group.

All in all, the appointment will take around 1 hour, and at the end you will leave with a shiny new folder with your maternity notes. This will be carried around by you pretty much always, and by the end of your pregnancy it will be a dog-eared representation of your nine-month whirlwind. I am told that some hospitals have entered the twenty-first century and done away with this paper folder, offering an app to access your pregnancy notes instead.

Rhesus disease

When you have your booking appointment for blood tests, you will be offered a blood group check. This tells the medical team if you are blood group A, B, AB or O, so that if anything happens that means you need a blood transfusion later, this information is all already documented. The test also tells us if you are rhesus positive or rhesus negative.

The rhesus factor is a protein found on the surface of red blood cells. If you are a rhesus-negative mother with a rhesus-positive baby, some of the baby's blood can cross into the mother's blood and sensitise the mother's immune system to the rhesus factor. If you are sensitised to the rhesus-positive blood, your immune system may then start to produce antibodies against the rhesus factor (anti-D antibodies), which can cross the placenta and attack the red blood cells of any subsequent rhesus-positive baby you carry. This can lead to a condition known as rhesus disease, in which the baby's red blood cells are destroyed, causing anaemia and other complications.

Therefore, if you are found to be rhesus negative at the booking appointment, your blood sample will be checked for anti-D antibodies. If you don't have these antibodies, you will be offered injections of anti-D immunoglobulin throughout your pregnancy, which helps to remove the rhesus foetal blood cells before they can cause sensitisation, to reduce the risk of developing an immune response to your baby's rhesus-positive blood.

If you already have developed the anti-D antibodies from a previous pregnancy, you will not be offered the anti-D immunoglobulin injections, as they won't help. Your pregnancy and baby will instead be monitored more closely. Your unborn baby may require a blood transfusion if they develop rhesus disease. After they are born, they are likely to be admitted to the neonatal unit, where they may have phototherapy treatment, blood trans-fusions and antibody injections.

Reassuringly, nowadays rhesus disease is uncommon, as we regularly test your rhesus status, and it is usually prevented early with the use of anti-D immunoglobulins.

WHAT TO LOOK OUT FOR – EARLY PREGNANCY SYMPTOMS

Some people are fastidious about their cycles, so within a day of missing their period they know they are pregnant. Others are more relaxed, or perhaps have irregular periods that can make knowing more difficult. However, there are often a few tell-tale signs that can alert even the most nonchalant woman to her impending pregnancy.

BREAST CHANGES

The surge of the hormones progesterone, oestrogen and prolactin in pregnancy boost blood flow to the breasts and cause changes in the tissue to prepare them for breastfeeding. This can result in them feeling more tender and swollen, similar to when you are on your period. You may also notice more veins overlying the breasts (I thought my boobs looked like they belonged to the Hulk for the majority of my pregnancy and during breastfeeding), and the nipples and the dark circle of skin around them (the areolae) can become darker. You can also notice the appearance of Montgomery glands, which are small, raised bumps on the areola. These are responsible for the lubrication of the nipple and antibacterial properties to limit breast and nipple infections.

FATIGUE

The fatigue is real. In my first trimester I was floored by an overwhelming tiredness that I had never experienced before. I was going to sleep at 7.30pm and would still wake up exhausted. There is a scene in the movie *The Wolf of Wall Street* where Leonardo DiCaprio's character has taken drugs called quaaludes, which are sedatives, and he has to drag himself out to his car, clawing his way across the floor in a semi-comatose state. Well, that was me for the first 12 weeks of my pregnancy. There are a number of reasons for this fatigue, including:

- Hormones – these play a big part in the fatigue of pregnancy, particularly progesterone, which surges in the first trimester. Progesterone is needed to help support the pregnancy and for milk production later on, and has a number of sleep-enhancing effects – it is essentially a sedative.
- Blood supply – to accommodate for the growing baby and placenta, your blood volume must increase, resulting in a lower blood pressure. Growing your placenta in itself is a mammoth task, and these increased demands on your body, together with a possible drop in blood sugar levels, may contribute to your fatigue.
- Anxiety – it is normal to feel anxious about a pregnancy, and with the fluctuation of hormones your emotional resilience may be low. These emotional changes often feed into your energy levels and your sleep.

What can you do to manage this fatigue? There are several options:

Do nothing – it will get better in the second trimester, though you will then hit the third trimester and your recurrent need to pee in the night, the 'you can't sleep on your back rule', back ache and reflux may all kick in (see page 37) and you become pretty sleep-deprived again. My advice would be to get as many baby-related chores and tasks done in the second trimester when you have a wave of energy again.

Eat well – I know this is easier said than done if you are suffering from nausea, in which case, just do what you can to survive. If you have not been hit too badly with nausea, do try to make some good food choices to support your body. Ensure you are eating enough fruits and vegetables, and that your meals are balanced with enough carbohydrates, proteins and healthy fats, avoiding processed foods where possible. Both you and your baby need more iron to make red blood cells whilst you're pregnant, therefore some pregnant women note that their iron levels drop, further aggravating the fatigue. Eating iron-rich foods may help; iron can be found easily in red meat and is also abundant in vegetables like dark green leafy vegetables, fortified cereals, pulses and nuts. However, our body is less able to absorb it in this vegetable form, so more of it needs to be consumed. To increase how much iron is absorbed from your food, eat these iron-rich foods alongside products high in vitamin C, like orange juice. You may find that eating little but often will help with maintaining your energy levels throughout the day.

Exercise – it may be a paradigm, but you need to expend energy to make energy. We know that exercising actually boosts your energy by increasing your blood flow and circulation, giving all your cells more oxygen, and by increasing your endorphin levels and giving you a little 'high'. Exercise improves your cardiovascular health and endurance, making everyday tasks less energy consuming.

Nap – make sleep a priority, aiming for early nights and the usual 7–9 hours of sleep each night[18], but, when needed, supplement your sleep with a nap. Understandably, some employers frown at naps in the middle of the office, especially if you have not revealed your pregnancy to them yet, in which case, just rest. Take the time during your lunch break to put your feet up, place your headphones on and close your eyes. This type of resting can still feel restorative even if you haven't managed to catch some zzzs. If you already have children, this type of restorative time can feel impossible to come by, as you are often stretched so thinly trying to entertain and keep safe your Tasmanian devil of a toddler. The constant and repetitive shouts of 'MUUUUUM' coming from the other room are not conducive to rest. I know how difficult it is, and I feel for you! This is a time when you really need your partner, friends or family to step up and grant you the space for rest.

Avoid caffeine – whilst caffeine may help beat the fatigue at that moment, its mean half-life (that is, the average time it takes for the concentration of caffeine in your body to decrease by half) is 5 hours[19], though this can range from anywhere between 1.5 hours and 9.5 hours, so, in those particularly susceptible, it can keep them awake at night. Not only that, but also it does cross the placenta, meaning the baby is also being kept awake, which may result in them being more active, kicking, poking and tapping away at your insides when you are trying to sleep, thus further compounding your fatigue.

INCREASED URINARY FREQUENCY

People often make the assumption that the need to pass urine frequently in pregnancy is due to the sheer weight of the womb on their bladder, which of course it can be in the later trimesters, but in the first trimester, when your bundle of joy is no bigger than a chia seed, there are other factors at play. It can mostly be put down to the surge in the hormones progesterone and human chorionic gonadotropin (HCG). The progesterone causes our smooth muscles (which is a type of muscle that contracts involuntarily), including those around the urethra, to relax, and the HCG causes an increased flow of blood to your pelvic area and kidneys. It is of course important to ensure that your urinary frequency is not being caused by a urinary tract infection (UTI), so do also look out for other symptoms including:

- Pain/burning on passing urine
- Blood in urine
- Cloudy urine
- Malodorous urine
- Abdominal pain
- Back pain
- Nausea or vomiting

MORNING SICKNESS

This is a misnomer, there is nothing 'morning' about it, it can affect you at any time of the day or night, though the symptoms can be worse in the mornings as your stomach is empty, having fasted through the night. I had the image of being an ethereal Earth Mother, feeding my child via my placenta with organic 'eat the rainbow' nutrients, chia and flaxseeds, and having a green goddess smoothie every morning, giving him/her the best start in life. The truth of the matter was I felt terribly nauseous, and the only thing I could eat for 12 weeks was cheese toasties. I would be woken by a wave of nausea at about 2am every night, and I would creep down to the kitchen to make a cheese toastie. Any attempt to make them 'healthy' by sneaking vegetables into them was heavily protested by my gut.

I think when we call it morning sickness, it implies to all the non-parents out there that it is a mild condition that you will overcome by 11am, when, in reality, in some cases it can be so severe that hospitalisation is required – a condition known as hyperemesis gravidarum (which occurs in between 0.3 and 3.6 per cent of pregnancies[20]). Morning sickness affects 80 per cent of pregnancies[21] but most often it subsides by weeks 16–20 of your pregnancy. I was incredibly lucky in that mine stopped at 12 weeks; one morning I just woke up from sleep and I didn't want to curl up around a toilet anymore.

Morning sickness occurs for several reasons, including the saliva in our mouths becoming more acidic in pregnancy, making foods and drinks taste less palatable. The acid in our stomach also becomes more acidic, which adds to the feeling of indigestion. Our gut motility is also slower in pregnancy, making us feel fuller and, due to the hormone relaxin, the muscle at the top of the stomach known as a sphincter becomes more relaxed, allowing the acid to travel up your oesophagus, causing nausea and vomiting. As if this wasn't enough, blood sugar levels become more erratic in pregnancy. In the first trimester your body utilises insulin more effectively, so your blood sugar levels can become slightly lower, which can also make you feel more nauseous.

So what can you do to ease morning sickness? A meta-analysis[22] reviewing 42 different studies about morning sickness, compared the outcomes of using acupuncture, chamomile, dimenhydrinate (an over-the-counter antihistamine used for motion sickness), doxylamine with vitamin B6 (a prescribed combination of antihistamine and vitamin B6), ginger, quince, metoclopramide (prescribed anti-sickness medication) and vitamin B6, against placebos. Of these different interventions, vitamin B6 and ginger had the best outcomes in terms of vomiting control and less-adverse events. The systematic review suggested there was only adequate evidence to support the use of ginger, and that even though favourable results were found for some of the other interventions, the strength of evidence for them was very low.

Ginger – this has been used in many cultures to aid digestion and morning sickness. It can be consumed in the form of teas, biscuits, capsules, drinks and candies. The evidence suggests that it may help with the symptoms of nausea, though it may not significantly reduce the frequency of vomiting[23]. As it does not pose any side-effects or adverse risks, it remains the first port of call for most pregnant women needing relief. The mode of action by which ginger gives us this anti-sickness property is still being unravelled, but it is thought to be a combination of how it increases the gastric tone and motility, and increased gastric emptying.

Acupressure – this is a type of massage based on Traditional Chinese Medicine, whereby pressure on certain points (acupoints) is thought to alleviate nausea. An easily accessed and classically utilised acupoint is the P6 point, which is found three fingers' breadth below the transverse crease of the inner wrist. There you can feel two tendons running vertically; the pressure point lies in between those tendons. Applying firm pressure there for 2–3 minutes is thought to relieve nausea. It is also possible to buy wristbands that consistently apply pressure to this point.

Medication – there are anti-sickness medications that can be given in pregnancy. Although these medicines (antihistamines and phenothiazines) are not specifically licensed for treating nausea and vomiting in pregnancy, their use is established in clinical practice and recommended by the Royal College of Obstetrics and Gynaecologists[24] for women whose symptoms have not responded to conservative management. Some prescribers and women may prefer the use of doxylamine/vitamin B6 because it is specifically licensed for use in pregnant women[25]. There is no evidence of harm from the use of the standard anti-sickness medications, though product literature for many of the medicines advises caution in pregnancy, so generally we try to limit medications in pregnancy where possible, and will weigh up the benefits against the risks. When the sickness could in itself be harming you (physically or emotionally) or the pregnancy, your doctor can prescribe them for you.

Food choices – even though you may not feel like it, please continue to eat regularly and avoid skipping meals. You may find that eating smaller meals more frequently is easier for your digestion, which can be as small and frequent as a mouthful every 15 minutes, if necessary. It is also easier to stomach carbohydrates than fatty foods, so keep it simple and try foods like crackers, pasta, toast and dry cereal, and place them by your bedside to have a nibble before you get up in the morning.

Hydration – becoming dehydrated can heighten the symptoms of nausea, so ensure you are regularly drinking. There is no 'ideal' amount to drink, as everyone's needs are different, and it can depend on your BMI, the weather, what foods you have been eating, how much you are vomiting, if you are sweating, etc. However, most people on average require around 1.5–2.5 litres of water a day (8–10 glasses)[26]. If you are struggling to drink, consider sucking on ice or an ice lolly, or drinking using a straw. For some, the smell/taste of chlorine in tap water can trigger nausea, so consider adding a slice of lemon or mint leaves, or drink cooled-down boiled water or mineral water instead.

Vitamin B6 – this is a water-soluble vitamin that is needed for a number of metabolic functions and for the development of our nervous system. It is found in many foods, including meat, fish, vegetables and bananas. It has been found that pregnancy (and taking oral contraception) can result in a deficiency of vitamin B6. How this vitamin works is not entirely understood, but it is thought that a deficiency may mean we do not produce the right amino acids needed to help reduce nausea. There have been studies that show an improvement in nausea scores in those who took this vitamin compared to women taking placebo[27]. The majority of studies, however, pertain to the use of vitamin B6 alongside doxylamine, but if you are looking for an over-the-counter option, some women choose to take vitamin B6 alone. In the UK, the Royal College of Obstetricians and Gynaecologists (RCOG) has not recommended the use of vitamin B6 as it states that there is a lack of consistent evidence, but in the US the American College of Obstetrics and Gynaecologists does recommend it in the treatment of nausea and vomiting in pregnancy[28].

When should you seek your doctor's help for morning sickness?

Whilst morning sickness is an accepted part of pregnancy, there is a point at which you should seek medical care. If it is severe enough that you have not been able to eat or drink for 24 hours, you are at risk of dehydration and malnutrition. Signs of dehydration include dark-coloured urine, not passing urine for over 8 hours, dizziness and feeling weak. In this situation you should speak to your GP, midwife or call NHS 111. This is also the case should your vomit become brownish or have blood in it. Sometimes urinary tract infections can be the cause of the increased vomiting in pregnancy, so should your vomiting symptoms come on rather suddenly, please also look out for the symptoms listed above under increased urinary frequency.

CRAVINGS

Everybody's cravings seem to be different; maybe you start to fancy mixing weird flavours together (bacon and cake anyone?) or eating foods you were not that bothered by pre-pregnancy. Or, in my case, not really eating much sweet stuff and only wanting to eat bread and cheese, and then eventually, when the morning sickness finished, adding in pickles of any variety. If it could be pickled, I wanted it. This lasted until my third trimester, when acid reflux put a firm stop to my desire for highly acidic foods. We often wonder whether pregnant women get these cravings to meet a nutritional deficit, for example, maybe your carnal desire to eat steaks is because you are iron-deficient, however, research suggests it is more complicated than that. It suggests that the foods most often craved are not the nutrient-dense ones, and that there may be more of a psychological basis to it[29]. Pregnancy is often a time when your cravings are not so harshly judged, so it may be that you are finally free to indulge in foods that you may otherwise feel guilty or embarrassed about eating. There is also the element of pregnancy being a difficult time, where the support of your loved one is paramount, and what can be more supportive than a midnight trek to McDonald's to buy you the strawberry milkshake that you otherwise could not live without?

BLOCKED NOSE

One in five pregnant women suffer with pregnancy rhinitis[30], which causes the feeling of a blocked or runny nose, like with a cold or hay fever. It can start in the first trimester but typically only becomes more noticeable in the second and third trimesters. It is thought to be caused by the effects of your pregnancy hormones, making the blood vessels and mucosa of the nose to swell up and become inflamed.

BLEEDING GUMS

Hormonal changes in pregnancy can cause your gums to be more susceptible to the effects of plaque and more swollen and inflamed. This is known as pregnancy gingivitis, and it can manifest with bleeding gums. Extra vigilance around dental hygiene is needed to help manage this. Remember that dental care is free on the NHS during pregnancy and for the first year after having a baby, so make use of this and see your dentist for a proper clean and advice on how to manage your gums.

EARLY PREGNANCY: A TIRED MAMMA'S SUMMARY

Choosing your hospital: you can generally give birth in either a labour ward, a birth centre or at home. On the NHS you need a referral to a hospital to begin your antenatal assessments and scans, which is usually done by self-referral, by going onto your chosen hospital's website and filling out a simple form.

The booking visit: your first appointment with your midwife, it's a chance to highlight any concerns you have about your pregnancy so the team can ensure you get the right antenatal support for your situation. You will be asked various questions, and your height, weight and blood pressure will be checked, and blood taken to test for three infections: HIV, hepatitis B and syphilis.

Rhesus disease: a condition in which a pregnant woman's immune system attacks her baby's red blood cells due to a mismatch in the blood type. Anti-D immunoglobulin injections can prevent the complications related to rhesus disease in a rhesus-negative mother carrying a rhesus-positive baby.

Early pregnancy symptoms: include breast changes, fatigue, increased urinary frequency, morning sickness and cravings. There are a number of lifestyle measures and supplements or medications to help manage these symptoms.

CHAPTER 3

PREGNANCY BE PREPARED

After the initial flurry of appointments, paperwork, rethinking your daily life and processing your news, it's time to establish a new way of living (for now!) to keep you in the best shape possible until the baby is born. That means thinking about what you can and can't eat for the health of your baby, as well as any lifestyle changes you will be advised to make, such as ensuring you are exercising safely for you pregnancy and getting enough sleep and rest when your body demands it.

FORBIDDEN FOODS

All this talk of cravings reminds me of all the forbidden foods that I promised myself I would eat by the truck load once I had birthed. It was a bit like being on the Island with Bear Grylls – food became an obsession. We spent an entire month sitting around the campfire talking about the foods we would eat the moment we left the Island. I distinctly remember one of my fellow islanders wanting a white baguette, with a thick pasting of salty butter and a cold chocolate bar in the middle. In retrospect, that sounds pretty basic, but at the time, when I was significantly undernourished, it was the primary thought getting me through (that and, of course, the thought of being reunited with my then fiancé, ahem!).

Simply put, when you are told you cannot have something, it is all you want. So read the following list at your own peril, with the knowledge that all you will want to eat from this page onwards is the following food! This list details which foods you are told to avoid during pregnancy as they can pose a risk to the developing baby:

CHEESE

This was a hard one for me. I am a cheese-board-for-dessert kind of woman. However, not all cheeses are off limits (hallelujah), only mould-ripened soft cheeses with white coatings around them (think Camembert and Brie), soft blue cheeses (think Roquefort and Gorgonzola), and any unpasteurised cheese/milk. This is because of the risk of a bacteria called listeria that can be found in these products, which can cause miscarriage and stillbirth. It is safe to eat these mould-ripened soft cheeses if they have been cooked until steaming hot as this kills off the bacteria.

FISH

Often hailed as a superfood, due to its omega 3 content, there are some limitations. Certain fish contain higher amounts of mercury, which can be harmful to unborn babies, so avoiding swordfish, marlin and shark is advisable. Even tuna is considered higher in its mercury content, so it is recommended that you limit tuna intake to two fresh steaks or four cans a week. Oily fish should also be limited to two portions a week, and this is because they have a higher concentration of pollutants in them. Oily fish include mackerel, salmon and herring. Raw shellfish is also on the no-no list, as they are higher risk for causing food poisoning. Most people assume that sushi is off the edibles list as it is also raw, however, you can have sushi if the fish has been frozen first.

MEAT

To complement your now very boring cheese board, you will also have a very lacking charcuterie board. This is because cold cured meats like prosciutto, salami and pepperoni have not been cooked in their preparation and therefore have an increased risk of containing the parasites that cause toxoplasmosis (see box, too). Whilst it is usually harmless, in pregnancy, toxoplasmosis can result in miscarriage, and if it does spread to your baby it can cause serious complications. For this same reason, it is advisable to eat your meat well done, with no blood or pink flesh. Eating game meat is also discouraged, as it can contain lead shot. Finally, pâté should be avoided, and this is for two reasons; first, often pâté is made with liver, which contains high amounts of vitamin A. Vitamin A in excess can cause congenital birth defects in your baby. Of course, this also means that avoiding eating liver itself is important. Secondly, pâté, including vegetarian pâté, can have a higher risk of listeria.

Pets and animals

If you have cats in your home, pregnant women should avoid contact with litter trays and cat faeces due to the risk of toxoplasmosis. They should also avoid any contact with sheep, cattle and goats who are pregnant or have recently given birth – so if you have other children who love to visit a petting zoo, take another adult along to assist with any feeding or petting and ensure your child and any other person who has contact with the animals thoroughly washes their hands, clothes and shoes before having contact with you[31, 32].

EGGS

If they have a red British Lion stamp on them, you can enjoy eggs all day long – raw, runny, hard. Heck, you can bathe in them. If they are not stamped, you can only eat them fully cooked, to reduce the risk of salmonella, which can cause food poisoning.

CAFFEINE

The thought of cutting out caffeine when you are already down on your pregnant, swollen and tired knees is frightening, but thankfully you don't have to omit it totally. Consuming high amounts of caffeine can lead to miscarriage and low-birth-weight babies, but the guidelines allow up to 200mg caffeine a day[33]. This amounts to two instant coffees (around 100mg each), two and a half cups of tea (around 75mg each) or five cans of coke (if you are having this many I fear for your gastro-intestinal tract!). Don't forget that even chocolate has caffeine, albeit small amounts; 50g of dark chocolate has around 25mg of caffeine.

WEIGHT IN PREGNANCY

A popular phrase from well-meaning parental figures is 'eat up, you're eating for two now', and whilst I need little excuse to delve into my MIL's fish pie and apple crumble for second helpings, unfortunately the saying is not quite true. Certainly your body's need for calories and nutrition does go up, but it does *not* double. While pregnancy is not the time to start a diet, you should be mindful of not gaining too much weight, as it can increase your risk of conditions like preeclampsia and gestational diabetes. Equally, though, not putting on enough weight may put you at risk of a preterm birth and low-birth-weight baby.

So, start as you mean to go on in your pregnancy. In the first and second trimesters, you do not need to eat any more than normal, it is only in the third trimester that you should eat around 200 calories per day more. It is worth reminding ourselves that 200 calories isn't actually that much. As an example, here are a few of my fave healthy snacks that come to around that:

- An apple with a tablespoon of peanut butter.
- Veggie crudites with two tablespoons of hummus.
- Half a pitta bread and a tablespoon of tzatziki.
- Small palmful of nuts.
- Fresh strawberries and pot of plain yoghurt.
- Half an avocado filled with a teaspoon of cottage cheese.

How much weight women put on during pregnancy can vary signif-icantly, as it can be affected by your pre-pregnancy weight and will obviously be higher in multiple pregnancies, but as a rule of thumb the NHS states most women will put on around 10–12.5kg. This weight gain will primarily occur in the second and third trimesters.

The Centers for Disease Control and Prevention (CDC) recommend the following weight gain as a guideline[34]:

Pre-pregnancy BMI	Weight gain – expecting one baby (kg)	Weight gain – expecting twins
underweight <18.5	12.7–18.1	22.7–28.2
normal 18.5–24.9	11.5–15.9	16.8–24.5
overweight 25–29.9	6.8–11.3	14–22.7
obese >30	5–9	11.3–19

The key to eating in pregnancy is to be kind to yourself, allow your midwife to track your weight during your appointments and be mindful of your intake but try not to be obsessive about it. Remember, the weight gain is not all body fat, and it is primarily made up of your baby, the placenta, the amniotic fluid, your breasts, the increased blood volume and natural fluid retention due to hormones.

EXERCISE IN PREGNANCY

There are numerous benefits to exercising during pregnancy, both for the expectant mother and the baby. So if you exercise regularly and are keen to continue to do so throughout your pregnancy, you should absolutely be encouraged to.

Exercise allows you to maintain your cardiovascular fitness and helps you manage your pregnancy weight and in turn reduce the risk of complications like gestational diabetes and high blood pressure. Exercising can also help strengthen the core muscles, alleviate pregnancy-prone back pain and prepare the body for labour. Exercises such as squats, lunges and resistance-band rows can be a great way to engage the deep core and prepare the body for an active labour. We also know that exercise can improve mood, anxiety and sleep, all of which can be impacted during pregnancy. The muscle strength and endurance afforded to you by exercising regularly may help you prepare for the physical demands of labour and delivery and aid in your postpartum recovery.

I was always frustrated when all I ever read about was pregnancy yoga and swimming. Both of these forms of exercise are beneficial, with pregnancy yoga helping flexibility, strength and relaxation, and swimming offering a low-impact, supportive full-body workout. However, if I'm honest, I found these both boring. I came from a flow and power yoga background, so staying centred and focused in the much gentler prenatal class was always challenging, and swimming was not my jam. Fortunately, most other forms of exercise are still considered safe. However, there are a few considerations you may need to make in certain sports:

Contact sports – any such sports that have a high risk of abdominal trauma should be avoided, for example, kickboxing, rugby or ice hockey. Having said this, I still attended boxing classes during pregnancy and teamed up with other pregnant women so that we would all be mindful of each other's bumps.

Exercising on your back – after the first trimester you should avoid any exercises that need you to be lying on your back. This is because of the pressure that this position puts on the blood vessels that supply the womb, which may reduce the blood flow. This limits certain exercises like abdominal crunches and leg lifts, but there are plenty of adaptations that you can make to still work these muscles without being on your back.

Overheating – evidence suggests that a body temperature greater than 39.2°C in the first trimester can slightly increase the risk of the baby having a birth defect[35]. It is unusual for our temperature to reach this without a fever or exercising in a hot climate before acclimatising. However, it is worth reconsidering hot yoga in the first trimester and taking it easy if you exercise in a hot climate. If you feel like you are getting hot, cool down, stay hydrated and take regular breaks.

Falls risk – be cautious with activities that have a high risk of falling and injury, like horse riding, skiing and bouldering. Your centre of gravity will change throughout pregnancy, making balance more difficult, so be mindful of this increased risk of falling.

Heavy weights – resistance training is still encouraged in pregnancy, as it helps to strengthen muscles, ease back pain, and improve posture and balance. But pregnancy is not the time to try to achieve personal bests, so focus more on your form over how many reps you complete or the weight you lift, to avoid injury.

Loose joints – during pregnancy the hormone relaxin is loosening your joints and ligaments, which can make you more prone to injury from over-extending your joints. Take this into consideration with any high-impact or fast movements.

Take it easy – when you need to rest, do. Your oxygen requirements go up when you are pregnant, and you might get out of breath faster than usual. Don't push yourself too hard, and rest if you find vigorous exercise more challenging.

Exercising to benefit your pregnant body

Shakira Akabusi, pre- and post-natal exercise specialist and founder of StrongLikeMum suggests:

'When it comes to exercise during pregnancy, we should not only consider what is safe but also what is most beneficial. For example, during the first trimester, where crunches and sit-ups are still considered "safe", they may not be the best choice, when considering what will best help to support your body throughout the next few months of pregnancy.

When exercising the core in pregnancy it's important that we look at all aspects of core function, including the surrounding muscles that will help to stabilise and realign our pelvis postpartum. Glute exercises such as squats, lunges, glute kickbacks and the bridge can be a fantastic way to work our glutes, which can help with our pregnancy posture and support postnatal recovery and pelvic realignment.

During pregnancy our pelvis is tilted forwards as the trimesters progress and the pregnancy bump grows. This shift can cause an increase of pressure onto the pelvic floor muscles, as the weight of internal organs shifts off the bony structures of the pelvis and rests more heavily onto the pelvic floor. This shift is natural and will largely come back into alignment itself around six months postpartum, however, it's important that we continue to work on glute exercises to support our posture, as well as deep core and pelvic floor movements to give our deep core muscles the support they need to manage this additional load. Exercises such as pelvic tilts, leg slides, the bridge and bird dog can be great to support the complete core.'

SLEEPING IN PREGNANCY

People say 'pregsomnia' or pregnancy-induced insomnia is your body's way of preparing you for the impending sleepless nights when the baby comes, but I can't think of any way that this would confer any medical advantage to entering parenthood. Starting your journey when you have no gas left in the tank is just a cruel joke.

Due to the increased fatigue that you develop in the first trimester, it is rarely a problem falling asleep, but 3am can become your new 6am. This is largely due to your pregnancy hormones (yes, those dreaded words rear their head again), which result in a number of effects:

Routine – progesterone's effect of excessive daytime sleepiness may be interrupting your usual sleep routines.

Snoring – progesterone can cause reduced muscle tone, which may mean you start snoring or develop sleep apnoea, which can wake you up through the night.

Congestion – inflammation of the nasal mucosa makes your nose feel blocked, like you have a permanent cold. It is thought to be caused by the hormones dilating the blood vessels and inflaming the mucous membranes in the nose. This nasal symptom may make it more difficult to breathe at night and can exacerbate the snoring.

Reflux – progesterone's effect on relaxing the valve between the stomach and oesophagus means that more acid can come up and cause discomfort. In addition, the growing womb puts upward pressure on the stomach, further pushing the acid up the oesophagus. Now try to lie down and sleep, and that acid is already at your throat!

Discomfort – between the bump, the bladder and the random aches, finding a comfortable position can be difficult. I found the most challenging part of this was the advice to avoid sleeping on your back (see 'Sleeping on your side' below). Investing in a pregnancy pillow can really help to relieve some of the discomfort, and it can then be used for nursing once the baby comes, so it has longevity. Although, I'd note that there was not enough room for me, bump, pillow AND husband in our bed, so naturally husband was demoted to a sofa bed.

Restless Leg Syndrome (RLS) – this is a condition that causes an overwhelming urge to move your legs. I suffer with it mildly anyway, but this ramped up massively in pregnancy, and research suggests that one in five pregnant women will experience it in their last trimester[36]. In some, RLS can also manifest as a crawling or creeping sensation to the lower limbs, or involuntary jerking. There are a number of theorised reasons behind the increased incidence in pregnancy, including deficiencies in folic acid and iron, and increases in oestrogen. Most of the medications ordinarily used to treat RLS cannot be used in pregnancy, so treatment is usually based on correcting any deficiencies and relieving symptoms when they come on. I spent a lot of evenings massaging my legs, stretching in yoga poses and going on 2am walks around my house. Other things that can help are hot baths, hot compresses and distraction techniques.

Anxiety – it's normal to feel worried – about the health of your baby, the nursery, work and finances, what labour has in store, 'Did I accidentally eat cured meat at the restaurant last night?', 'When is the last time I can get a wax before labour?', 'When should I pack my hospital bag', etc. These anxieties can be hard to park in the middle of a quiet night, and they may stop you from falling back to sleep. Try keeping a notepad next to your bed and write these thoughts down so that you can re-visit them in the morning rather than ruminate overnight. If your anxieties seem to be getting the better of you, do speak to your doctor about them.

SLEEPING ON YOUR SIDE

The advice of the NHS is to sleep on your side from 28 weeks (third trimester) of pregnancy due to the increased risk of stillbirth by lying on your back[37]. The first trial that made a link between the risk of stillbirth and the mother's sleeping position was a New Zealand Study carried out in 2011, which showed a nearly four-fold risk of harm to your baby by sleeping on your back[38]. As it was the first study to report maternal sleep-related practices as a risk factor for stillbirth and it was a small study, it called for urgent confirmation in further studies. A further study in Australia confirmed that sleeping on your back was an additional risk factor for stillbirth in an already compromised foetus[39]. But, again, it was a small study, and it was not until the results of the fourth and largest study at that point, The Midlands and North of England Stillbirth Study (MiNESS[40]), were published, that pregnant women in their third trimester were advised to sleep on their side. This study asked women who had a late pregnancy stillbirth about their sleeping habits and it found that women who go to sleep lying on their back have a 2.3-fold increased risk of late pregnancy stillbirth. In the UK, devastatingly, one in 225 pregnancies end in stillbirth[41], and it was estimated by this study that if all pregnant women in the UK went to sleep on their side in the third trimester there would be a 3.7 per cent decrease in stillbirth, saving 130 babies' lives a year.

WHY DOES POSITION MAKE A DIFFERENCE?

The reason is still unknown. What we do know is that studies have shown that when a pregnant woman lies on her back, the baby becomes less active and there are changes in its heart rate[42]. It is believed this could be related to the pressure that the combined weight of the baby and womb puts on the main blood vessels that supply the womb while lying on your back, which may reduce the blood flow, and therefore oxygen delivery, to the baby.

DOES IT MATTER IF YOU LIE ON YOUR LEFT OR RIGHT SIDE?

The current advice is that you can lie on either side, though there have been some suggestions to favour your left side. In theory, the 'left-sided rule' could make sense because it allows for optimal flow from a large vein called the inferior vena cava (IVC), which runs on your right side, carrying blood to your heart and your baby. Other organs that feel relieved from lying on your left side are your liver (which is positioned on the right) and the kidneys, which drain into the IVC. This better functioning of your kidneys may help alleviate pregnancy swelling in your hands and feet.

However, several studies have not found any difference in risk between sleeping on the right or left side[43], so the advice still remains unchanged that you can sleep on either side. In addition to reducing your risk of stillbirth, side sleeping may also promote healthy spine alignment, reduced acid reflux and snoring.

WHAT IF YOU WAKE IN THE NIGHT ON YOUR BACK?

Don't panic, it's normal to move around in your sleep. When we go to sleep we tend to spend the longest period of time in that same position in the night, and your huge bump in the third trimester is likely to be uncomfortable enough to stop you from sleeping on your back for too long anyway. If you are struggling with the side sleep, place a pillow between your legs, as it helps align your pelvis and makes it more comfortable. You can also place a pillow behind your back to stop you from rolling over in the night. I found it helpful to tie a bun at the back of my head, which would just stop me from comfortably sleeping on my back. If you don't have long hair to do this, I've heard of people sewing a tennis ball to the back of their PJ tops to stop the roll back. If you do wake up on your back, just roll back onto your side and continue your slumber.

GOING PUBLIC – WHEN TO TELL YOUR FRIENDS AND FAMILY

You are pregnant, you're so excited, you want to shout it from the rooftop, but then you are suddenly gripped by anxiety. Who do you tell first, when do you tell them? Instagram said I need to do a gender reveal cake/balloon, what even is that?

Sharing your news is a deeply personal and often culturally influenced decision, but many people choose to wait until the 12-week mark to tell their nearest and dearest, as this is the point at which risk of miscarriage falls. Sadly, 10–25 per cent of pregnancies end in miscarriage[44], but around 80 per cent of these occur in the first trimester. When you break it down further, after 12 weeks, the risk of miscarriage falls to 5 per cent for the rest of the pregnancy.

Some people just want to wait until they hear the baby's heartbeat for the first time, or once they have had an ultrasound scan. Perhaps previous miscarriages may also determine when you feel comfortable telling people. Or maybe the right time for you is when your bump starts showing, but truly there is no hard-and-fast rule about when to tell people, you need to do what is comfortable for you.

It is important to recognise that in traditionally waiting to tell people only after you are past those early weeks, you can potentially be robbing yourself of much-needed support should a miscarriage occur. Miscarriage is a sensitive and emotionally challenging experience that often requires compassion, understanding and support, yet there is still stigma around it. The lack of open conversation around miscarriage in society further propagates this stigma, making people feel like they are the only ones going through it, therefore making them even less likely to speak out.

So don't feel confined to keeping this wonderful news hidden from the world if you don't want to, or consider who you want to have by your side in case of complications or emotional support and then share the news with these selected friends and family early on to provide a strong support system.

Personally, I found the secrecy around early pregnancy difficult to manage. I pretended to drink a G+T when actually I'd enlisted the help of the waiter on my trip to the loo to make it just a T, but not to mention that to anyone on the table. Being that annoying friend who only wanted to meet between the times of 12pm and 6pm, because before 12 I was still a mess from the tumultuous night's sleep and nausea, and after 6pm I was comatose, but I couldn't tell anyone why. Or instantly regretting organising a GoApe session for my best friend's Hen do, when I found out that it is not recommended in pregnancy and spending the entire time freaking out that if I went, I'd miscarry. All this, whilst knowing that most miscarriages are caused by factors beyond a mother's control, like chromosomal abnormalities, which means the baby doesn't develop properly. Even though I am a GP, armed with the facts and the science, the fear of the unknown that came along with being a new mother was still very much there. For me, I felt the overwhelming need to have my ultrasound scan first before telling anyone, so until 12 weeks it was just myself and my husband who were privy to this special news. Despite the difficulty in keeping it confidential, there was something lovely about this plum-sized blob being our little secret.

YOUR BABY'S GROWTH

You see your tummy expanding, you feel all of the new symptoms, but what is actually happening inside you at each of the trimesters? It is absolutely fascinating when you start to understand the remarkable changes that are happening under your very nose. Your baby's growth is testament to the intricate marvel that is unfolding within your womb.

How big is your baby?

My book is mainly science, but I decided to add this in, because, in truth, this was my most-googled question throughout my pregnancy! Every week without fail, I wanted to know what fruit-size equivalent my growing foetus was.

Week	Size
3–4	Poppy seed
5	Sesame
6	Grain of rice
7	Blueberry
8	Raspberry
9	Grape
10	Date
11	Fig
12	Plum
13	Kiwi
14	Peach
15	Pear
16	Avocado
17	Orange
18	Pomegranate
19	Grapefruit
20	Mango
21	Cantaloupe
22–24	Aubergine
25–28	Papaya
29–32	Butternut squash
33–36	Honeydew
37–40	Watermelon

FIRST TRIMESTER

This is the period that spans from conception to the end of week 12, and it is when your foetus grows rapidly from a single fertilised cell to a multicellular organism.

Weeks 1–4 – your pregnancy is dated from the first day of your last period, so in the first couple of weeks you aren't *actually* pregnant, only preparing for it. We are harping back to school biology class, but it all begins simply when the sperm fertilises the egg to form a zygote, with a full set of chromosomes. Over the next few days, the zygote divides several times to form a blastocyst. The inner group of this rapidly dividing ball of cells becomes the embryo and the outer group becomes the cells that provide nourishment. At around days 10–14 after conception, this blastocyst implants by attaching itself to the womb lining. And so your pregnancy begins. The embryo develops within the amniotic sac, and the outer layer of this sac will develop into the placenta. The cells from this outer layer are already starting to root into the wall of the womb to establish a rich blood supply. In the first 4 weeks of pregnancy you are unlikely to notice many symptoms other than a missed period, though on implantation, you might have symptoms like spotting and cramping.

Weeks 5–8 – your embryo's major organs start to form, including the brain, liver, kidneys, spine and tiny tube-like heart, which begins to beat. The baby's limb buds (which will become arms and legs) also begin to emerge. The outer layers of the embryo's cells fold to form a hollow tube known as the neural tube, which will eventually become the brain and spinal cord. You are taking folic acid to prevent defects in the formation of this tube. By week 8 your embryo becomes upgraded to a foetus. It is around the 7–8-week mark that you might notice symptoms of pregnancy, like fatigue, passing urine more frequently, breast tenderness and morning sickness.

Weeks 9–12 – growth rapidly continues, with more intricacies forming, like facial features including the eyes, ears and nose. The fingers and toes also become more defined, with fingernails forming, and the nervous system develops further forming reflexes. The heart is now fully formed and your placenta develops fully, allowing for efficient nutrient exchange. By 12 weeks your foetus has all its organs, muscles and bones in place. Your body is having to adapt to make room for this growing foetus, and you might notice some cramping, bloating and constipation.

SECOND TRIMESTER

This includes weeks 13 to 27 and is often referred to as the 'golden period' of pregnancy. Most of the unpleasant symptoms have gone, and your baby is continuing to grow and refine.

Weeks 13–16 – your baby will be moving, but you may not feel it yet. Their sensory organs are also beginning to develop, so they now have taste buds and can start to hear. They are able to put these taste buds into practice as they begin to swallow small amounts of amniotic fluid. This will get their stomachs and kidneys functioning. They will start hearing your voice and heartbeat, so get chatting to them! They are getting their own unique fingerprints, and they are growing a soft fine hair (lanugo) over their body, as well as a protective waxy coating called vernix. Their ovaries/testes have developed within their bodies. With your negative pregnancy symptoms waning you might start to notice an increase in libido with the increase of blood flow to your pelvic area alongside the fluctuations in hormones.

Weeks 17–20 – as your baby grows, you may start to feel their movements, initially as little flutters, or 'is that just some gas?' type bubbling, but soon enough it becomes unmistakable. Their hair grows and nails begin to form. Their reproductive systems are developing, becoming externally obvious, allowing radiologists to identify gender on scans. Their eyes can move but they still keep them shut, though they may be able to differentiate between bright lights shining at your tummy.

Weeks 21–27 – the baby starts to put on weight and grow more now, they have eyelids that can open and close, and their lungs are maturing to prepare for breathing. With the increase in your baby's weight over this second trimester you will start to look 'properly' pregnant and may develop backache. Your skin will stretch to accommodate the bigger bump and this may result in stretch marks. The hormonal changes may also mean your breasts start leaking some milk, and the relaxation of the veins in the pelvis can result in piles.

THIRD TRIMESTER

This is the final stretch, from week 28 up to birth.

Weeks 28–32 – your baby's brain is growing and developing and they are refining reflexes like sucking and swallowing. Your partner can sometimes even hear the baby's heartbeat if they put their ear against your tummy. The baby's lanugo and vernix might start to disappear. Space is getting tighter, and you might experience acid reflux and increasing breathlessness. It is also more common to start having leg cramps at this stage of pregnancy, though it is not clear why.

Weeks 33–36 – their immune system is becoming more advanced, and their bones are hardening, with the exception of the skull, which stays soft to aid the passage through the birth canal. Most babies will be lying head down ready for birth by this point, but don't worry if they haven't got into this position yet, they can still turn (or be turned!). If you are having a boy their testes will be making their descent from the abdomen into their scrotum. You will probably find yourself slowing down now, though trying to keep active can help through labour. You may start to feel Braxton Hicks contractions, which feel like tightening or contractions, as a practice for labour.

Weeks 37–birth – this is considered full term and your baby is ready to be born. Their lungs have matured, ready for breathing, and their digestive tract is also fully formed ready to feed. The baby is more likely to move down into the birth canal – known as engaging. Whilst it can feel like a pressure in the pelvic area, it can relieve some of the upper abdominal symptoms like heartburn/reflux and you feel like you can take deeper breaths.

12-WEEK SCAN

Your first scan, sometimes known as your dating scan, or your 12-week scan, usually occurs between 10 and 14 weeks. Its primary purpose is to:

- Estimate when your baby will be due, based on its size.
- See how many babies you are having.
- Check on its development.
- Assess its position.
- Assess the position of your placenta.

If you choose to, you can also have the nuchal translucency scan at this appointment, which is part of the screening test for Down's syndrome, Edwards' syndrome and Patau's syndrome (see antenatal screening tests on page 50 for more information). This scan uses ultrasound, which are sound waves, to build up a picture of your baby. It's painless and has no known side-effects to mother or baby. You will usually be asked to drink water before the appointment so that your bladder is full, as this helps get a better image. Then you will lie back on the bed whilst the ultrasonographer uncovers your tummy (I'd recommend wearing loose clothing so you're not struggling to expose yourself in your bodycon number) and puts unreasonably cold gel onto it. He or she then smears it around with the ultrasound probe to get the best views of your baby and may have to put light pressure on certain areas. The pressure can sometimes feel a bit firmer or uncomfortable, especially when your bladder is full, or if the baby is in an awkward position and the probe has to go over the same area multiple times, but you can ask the ultrasonographer to pause if it is too uncomfortable.

The whole appointment usually takes around 20 to 30 minutes. My husband attended this appointment with me as it was just before Covid struck, and having seen a million ultrasounds in the past, I expected to feel fairly matter of fact about it, but within moments of hearing the heartbeat, I squeezed his hand and a tear rolled down.

Whilst there is currently no evidence to suggest that this scan is unsafe or that there are grounds for questioning its safety, it is suggested that any non-medical scans are avoided in the first 10 weeks. Even though early scans are often desired by parents who want to confirm the pregnancy by ultrasound, we know that in this period up to 10 weeks the embryo is potentially more vulnerable at this early stage and would be most susceptible to any perturbation.

Although this scan is often a happy one where you finally get that little black and white photo of your baby looking like a small alien, or, as in my case, a disconcerting parrot (note, your hospital may charge for these, so take money/card just in case), please do be prepared that in a small number of cases this scan can also uncover some abnormalities. Remember, you do not have to have this scan if you do not want it and if finding out about these abnormalities would make no difference to your plans, some choose not to go ahead with it. However, even if it makes no difference to your plans and you would continue with the pregnancy irrespective of the outcome, we know that earlier detection of some conditions can allow for better management of any pregnancy complications relating to it.

Please note that what this 12-week scan does NOT do in the UK is tell you the gender of your baby. Whilst this scan can theoretically predict the gender based on the angle of the genital tubercle, which is the precursor of the penis and clitoris (vertically up for boy, flat or down for girl), this is not something offered on the NHS in the UK. This is because, first, it is not the most reliable predictor at this stage in the pregnancy, but also knowing the gender at this stage may encourage some people to have a termination purely because the baby's gender isn't what they hoped, for myriad reasons. If you decide you want to know the sex of your baby, you will be able to find out at the anomaly scan at around 20 weeks of pregnancy. You can also have a private scan to find out sooner.

ANOMALY SCAN

The anomaly scan, also known as the 20-week scan, is another ultrasound scan that usually takes place between 18 and 21 weeks of pregnancy. Its purpose is to check on the development of your baby and it looks in detail at their brain, heart, spinal cord, kidneys, bowels and limbs. Some conditions are easier to detect on than others, for example, spina bifida is picked up on this scan in 90 per cent of cases[45], however, heart defects are only spotted 50 per cent of the time[46]. The scan screens for the following 11 conditions:

- Anencephaly
- Open spina bifida
- Cleft lip
- Diaphragmatic hernia
- Gastroschisis
- Exomphalos
- Serious cardiac abnormalities
- Bilateral renal agenesis
- Lethal skeletal dysplasia
- Edwards' syndrome
- Patau's syndrome

If the ultrasonographer picks up that your baby is at higher risk of a chromosomal condition, you will then be offered a diagnostic test. You can also ask for the baby's gender at this scan.

Pros and cons of finding out your baby's sex

Personally, I chose not to find out about the sex of my baby. I felt I had so few genuine and exciting surprises in my otherwise very regimented life, that I wanted to keep this as one of them. I also hoped that by leaving it unknown, at the final stages of labour, it might give me the impetus to push that little harder! I remember at the 20-week ultrasound scan being asked if we wanted to know the gender and we both said no. We had both, for some reason, assumed that it was a girl, and we named her 'Chia', as that was the size she was when we found out about the pregnancy. At the scan, they told us to look away at the point at which the ultrasonographer was examining the genitalia, but with my doctor hat on I thought I had glimpsed his little testicles. I never told Rupert and, to be honest, by the time the baby came, we had referred to it as a girl so much that I had entirely ignored and forgotten what I had possibly seen on the scan!

Other pros and cons include:

Pros	Cons
You can have a gender reveal party – think gender-revealing balloons, cakes, fireworks!	You can have a baby shower instead, or have a naming party, or a meet and greet party. Lots of excuses for parties!
You only have to think of one name. Halving the colossal effort of name-choosing is a relief.	The ultrasounds are not always right, so you may end up preparing everything for a certain gender only to have a shock at the birth.
You can plan for gender-appropriate clothes and nursery, if that appeals to you.	Who cares about gender-appropriate colours? Harris wore a pink flowery onesie and glittery unicorn hat for most of his infancy. He didn't care, so I didn't care.
When pregnancy and labour feels a little out of control with a lot of unknowns, this is one thing you can know. It may therefore give you a slight sense of calm.	You get to hear about people's strange ways of predicting sex. I had heard Holly Willoughby had a 100 per cent success rate in predicting gender, so whilst I was on *This Morning*, after my segment was done, I asked her theory on my baby bump. She looked at my bump, lay her hand on either side of it, and said 'boy'.

Pros	Cons
It gives you time to come to terms with the gender, especially if you were hoping for a different outcome.	The surprise is really fun.
You might feel a bit more connected to your baby whilst you carry it if you think you know a bit more about it.	There's so much more to learn about your little one than the gender.

ANTENATAL SCREENING TESTS

In addition to the ultrasound screening tests you may also be offered blood tests to detect for early signs of complications.

BLOOD TESTS

Thalassaemia and sickle cell disease are both inherited blood conditions that affect the way red blood cells carry oxygen around the body. All pregnant women are offered screening blood tests to look for these conditions. The test does not screen the baby, but if we find that the mother is a carrier of either of these conditions, we can then screen the father. If he too is found to be a carrier of one of these conditions, then you will be offered screening tests for the baby.

You will also be offered screening for the infectious diseases HIV, hepatitis B and syphilis. HIV is a virus that affects your immune system, and can be passed to your baby through childbirth and breast-feeding, however, if you are aware of your status you will be offered antiviral medication that significantly reduces the risk of passing it on. Furthermore, you will be offered safer ways of delivering and feeding the baby, as well as medication for the baby to reduce the risk that they will contract the virus. Similarly, hepatitis B can also be passed on to the baby through birth, but if we are aware of the infection beforehand, the baby will be offered a hepatitis B immunisation at birth to protect them from getting it. Syphilis can be easily treated with antibiotics, but left untreated it can cause harm to the unborn baby.

COMBINED TESTS

The combined tests are so-called because they combine the findings of the ultrasound scans and the blood tests, to assess the risk of your baby having Down's syndrome, Edwards' syndrome and Patau's syndrome. The blood test is often taken at the same time as your 12-week scan. At the 12-week scan they will assess the nuchal translucency (NT), which is a measurement of the fluid under the skin at the back of the baby's neck. The measurement increases with the baby's gestational age (how many weeks pregnant you are), but the higher the measurement compared to babies with the same gestational age, the higher the risk is for these conditions. The combined test results and the mother's age are input into an algorithm which gives us the risk of your baby having any of these conditions. The results will come back as either 'lower risk', which means you have a risk of less than 1 in 150, or 'higher risk', where the risk is higher than 1 in 150. If your results show that your baby is at higher risk, you will be offered non-invasive prenatal testing (NIPT) and diagnostic tests. The NIPT is another, more accurate screening blood test and may help you decide whether or not to pursue the diagnostic test. The diagnostic tests include amniocentesis and chorionic villus sampling (CVS), and as the name suggests they are used to make a diagnosis.

During an amniocentesis, a long needle is inserted through the abdominal wall to the amniotic sac, with the guidance of ultrasound, and a small sample of the amniotic fluid is taken. The CVS involves a small sample of cells being taken from the placenta. This can be done either through a needle through the abdomen, or less commonly by using forceps inserted through the cervix. Some may choose to have the NIPT first, or indeed decline the diagnostic tests altogether, because, unfortunately, there is a risk of miscarriage with both the amniocentesis and CVS of around 0.5–1 per cent[47]. As there is no cure for these conditions, careful consideration needs to be made as to whether you would like to have these tests done and what you will do with the results. Some will choose to continue their pregnancy, others will choose to end it.

QUADRUPLE BLOOD SCREENING

If it was not possible to do the nuchal translucency screen at the 12-week scan because of the position of the baby, or because you are more than 14 weeks pregnant, you will be offered a quadruple blood screening instead, between 14 and 20 weeks of pregnancy. This, however, can only test for Down's syndrome and is not as accurate at the combined test.

VACCINATIONS

Your body is incredible, and it adapts in so many ways to keep your unborn baby safe. One of these adaptations is your immune system, which needs to be modified to ensure that it does not reject the baby as a 'threat'. This may, however, leave you more vulnerable to other infections, which is why you are often labelled as being 'immunocompromised' if you are pregnant, and certain vaccinations are therefore recommended.

Flu – in addition to your immunocompromise, when you are pregnant your ability to take in big and full breaths can be limited by your enormous bump, and this can put you at increased risk of developing pneumonia and complications should you pick up the flu. Your baby can also be affected by the flu, resulting in premature births, low birth weights and even deaths in some rare and tragic cases. The flu vaccine is the best protection we have against this virus, and it is best to get it in the autumn, before the flu season really kicks off.

Whooping cough – this is actually a vaccination to protect your baby, as the antibodies from the vaccine pass to your baby through the placenta, offering some protection against whooping cough until they are able to have their own vaccine when they are 8 weeks old (see vaccination schedule on page 274).

We worry about whooping cough in newborns, as they are at the greatest risk of severe illness from it. The best time to have this vaccine is between 16 and 32 weeks pregnant, though you can have it right up until labour if necessary.

Covid-19 – unfortunately the pandemic has brought an additional recommended vaccine to pregnant women. You are at higher risk of complications from Covid-19 if you are pregnant, and contracting this virus in your third trimester could also put your baby at harm. The vaccination may offer your baby some antibodies too. The guidelines are changing constantly, so it is important to keep an eye out for the government recommendations, but currently they are offering additional autumn/winter boosters to pregnant women. With new variants in circulation, it is advised that pregnant women have the full course of vaccines, which includes the two initial doses and the booster as this makes you 88 per cent less likely to be admitted to hospital with Covid than those who are unvaccinated[48].

GLUCOSE TOLERANCE TEST

You may be invited to have a glucose tolerance test (GTT). This procedure assesses how well you process sugar and it is used to diagnose gestational diabetes mellitus (GDM). GDM is a type of diabetes that occurs in pregnancy and is characterised by high blood sugar levels. It usually develops from around the 24th week of pregnancy, when the body's demand for insulin increases due to the growing placenta and the hormones it produces. Insulin is a hormone that our pancreas produces to regulate blood sugar levels, but in GDM the body may not produce enough insulin or cannot use it effectively, resulting in elevated blood sugar levels.

GDM can affect your pregnancy in a number of ways. It can lead to your baby growing larger than usual, jaundice, too much amniotic fluid, premature birth, pre-eclampsia and, in rare cases, stillbirth.

Certain factors can put you at an increased risk of GDM, and if you have any of these risk factors you will be invited to have a GTT, at around 26–28 weeks of pregnancy. The risk factors include:

- Age >40
- BMI >30
- Previous gestational diabetes
- Family history of diabetes – one of your parents or siblings
- Previous baby >4.5kg at birth
- Ethnicity with a high prevalence of diabetes, including South Asian, Black, African-Caribbean or Middle Eastern
- History of gastric bypass or other weight-loss surgery

The procedure involves fasting from midnight the previous night, then having a blood test in the morning. You are then given a drink with a specific amount of glucose in it, rest, and 2 hours later you repeat this blood test to assess how your body is processing this glucose. This isn't the most fun test to have – you are a hungry pregnant woman sitting in a heaving waiting room, with huge delays to your appointment, being bled twice in 2 hours, and you aren't allowed to leave the hospital in that time, all of which is a recipe for disaster in my books. On the plus side, the drink tastes like a Capri-Sun, which I haven't had in decades, and the nostalgia put a smile on my face!

If you are diagnosed with GDM, you will be given advice about diet and physical activity to manage your blood sugar levels. If lifestyle measures are not enough to control the blood sugar, you will also be treated with medication. As GDM puts you at increased risk of developing type 2 diabetes after you have given birth, you should also have a blood test 6–13 weeks postnatally and then annually thereafter if the result was normal.

PREGNANCY COMPLICATIONS

Pregnancy is often a celebrated and transformative journey, but there is a diverse set of challenges that can arise along the way. These potential complications can occur from the early stages to the final moments of pregnancy. Although the thought of complications during this delicate time can cast shadows on what should be a miraculous period, it is always best to be informed about the signs and symptoms in case you experience any of them, so that you can get prompt treatment and healthier outcomes.

DEEP VEIN THROMBOSIS (DVT)

A deep vein thrombosis (DVT) is a blood clot that forms in a deep vein within the leg, calf or pelvis. The concern with a DVT is that it can break off and start travelling through the veins to other parts of the body where it might get lodged. If it gets lodged in the lungs it is known as a pulmonary embolism (PE) and this can require emergency attention. Pregnancy increases your risk of developing a DVT, though you are at your highest risk immediately after giving birth. They occur in one or two in 1,000 women during pregnancy or the first 6 weeks postnatally[49]. The symptoms of a DVT include pain, swelling and tenderness to your leg (usually your calf but can also be the thigh), which can also look red and feel hot to the touch.

The treatment of DVT is heparin, which is an injected blood thinner. Heparin does not cross the placenta, so it will not affect your baby. If you think you are going into labour, you will be advised by your midwife/doctor to stop taking the heparin injections. An epidural will not be able to be given until 24 hours have passed since your last injection, so alternative pain relief may need to be discussed. If you are having a Caesarean section within that 24-hour window, the surgery will need to be carried out under general anaesthetic.

HIGH BLOOD PRESSURE

Gestational hypertension is high blood pressure that is diagnosed in pregnancy, typically after 20 weeks, which returns to normal within 6 weeks of having your baby. It is defined as a blood pressure reading of greater than 140/90 and affects about four to eight in 100 pregnancies[50]. However, between two and eight in 100 pregnant women then go on to develop pre-eclampsia. This can be a serious condition whereby you have high blood pressure and protein in your urine. It is usually mild and has no effect on the pregnancy or baby, but in rare cases it can be severe, affecting your organs, blood clotting and possibly progressing to seizures (in one in 4,000 pregnancies). It could also affect how your baby grows. In both gestational diabetes and pre-eclampsia, you will be monitored, and you may be offered medication to bring down the blood pressure. In pre-eclampsia, you may have more regular scans to check on your baby's growth, and you may be advised to have your baby earlier (usually by 37 weeks), which may mean an induction or a Caesarean section.

INTRAHEPATIC CHOLESTASIS

Intrahepatic cholestasis of pregnancy (ICP) is a liver condition that can develop in pregnancy. It occurs when the bile acid, which usually travels from your liver to your gut, does not flow correctly and builds up instead. The main symptom is an itch without a rash, which tends to occur in the third trimester. In rare cases some women also become jaundiced. It affects around seven in 1,000 women in the UK, though it is more common in women of South Asian descent (where the figure is fifteen in 1,000)[51]. The itch tends to be very distressing and will only resolve upon giving birth. There is an increased chance that your baby will pass meconium before they are born (see 'What can go "wrong" in labour?' on page 108 for information about meconium), that they are born prematurely and, if you have severe ICP, your risk of stillbirth is increased to 3 per cent[52]. As this increased risk of stillbirth usually occurs after 36 weeks of pregnancy, you may be advised to have your baby sooner, at 35 weeks.

HYPEREMESIS GRAVIDARUM

This is a condition of extreme sickness in pregnancy. It affects one to three in 100 pregnancies[53] and is defined as nausea and vomiting that is so severe that it leads to dehydration and weight loss. Should you be unable to tolerate any fluids, you might be admitted to hospital for treatment, where the midwife or doctor will also assess your urine for signs of dehydration, check your bloods and assess for any weight loss. You are likely to be given fluids through an IV line, as well as anti-sickness medication and vitamin B1 (thiamine). You may also be advised to wear compression stockings and to have heparin injections to reduce your risk of a DVT, which is more likely if you are immobile and dehydrated. Once you can start eating and drinking more, you will be discharged with oral medication. Hyperemesis gravidarum is unlikely to affect your baby, though you may have a baby with a lower-than-expected birth weight in severe cases.

UNEXPECTED BLEEDING

You're living your best pregnant life (omitting nausea, fatigue, breast tenderness, anxiety and random rages), happily wearing your 'baby on board' badge and stroking your tummy, when one day you sit on the toilet and you see a streak of blood on the tissue paper. Your heart sinks into what feels like a neverending cavernous hole. It happened to me at around 9 weeks of pregnancy, and it's nigh on impossible not to think the worst. At the time, I tried to be nonchalant about it, convincing myself that it was 'fine' because it was so early on and miscarriage is so common. But that was just my brain's way of trying to protect myself. It's not fine; it's terrifying, though, thankfully, my bleeding was not caused by a miscarriage.

A miscarriage is defined as when a pregnancy ends before 24 weeks, and, sadly, one in five pregnancies ends this way[54]. The majority of miscarriages occur in the first 12 weeks of pregnancy and this is often because there is something wrong with how the baby is developing. It is natural to wonder if there was something you could have done differently to prevent it, and in the vast majority of cases the answer is no, there was nothing you could have done to change that outcome.

In addition to bleeding, other symptoms of a miscarriage can include abdominal pain and cramping, and resolution of pregnancy symptoms, like breast tenderness and nausea. There are, however, a number of reasons why one can bleed in pregnancy which don't mean you are losing the pregnancy.

Causes of bleeding in early pregnancy (up to 12 weeks):

Implantation – once the egg is fertilised, the embryo beds itself down into the nice cosy wall of the womb, and on implant it can cause some spotting. This type of bleeding tends to occur early on, usually at around the time that a period would be expected, so it can sometimes throw people off the scent of their pregnancy, assuming this bleeding was just a 'light' period. It is often just a light pink or brown bleed that stops within 1 or 2 days.

Cervical changes – pregnancy hormones make the cervix softer and richer with blood flow. This can mean that it is more likely to bleed, especially after sex, but this will not cause harm to your pregnancy.

Infection – infections like thrush or sexually transmitted infections can cause inflammation of the cervix or vagina, which can result in bleeding. If an infection is found, you will be prescribed medication accordingly, and your partner may also need to be treated.

Chorionic haemorrhage – this is what I had, and it occurs when the placenta partially detaches from where it was implanted on the wall of your womb. This causes a blood clot (haematoma) to develop between the membrane surrounding the embryo (the chorion) and the wall of the womb. This condition can be diagnosed by the clot being seen on an ultrasound scan. Most of these clots resolve themselves with no issue, but there are some rare cases in which the placenta separates from the womb wall, increasing the risk of miscarriage or premature labour.

Threatened miscarriage – this is when you experience bleeding and abdominal pain but you do not go on to lose the pregnancy, and a heartbeat remains.

Causes of bleeding in later pregnancy:

Cervical changes – as detailed above, this is also relevant in later pregnancy.

Infection – as detailed above, this is also relevant in later pregnancy.

Show – this is a pink, jelly-like substance known as a 'mucus plug'. The mucus comes away from the cervix as it starts to open and is a sign that labour is about to start.

Low-lying placenta – this occurs when your placenta attaches low down in your womb, sometimes wholly covering your cervix (known as placenta praevia), and can cause heavy bleeding, usually in the last 3 months of pregnancy. The low-lying placenta often grows up and out of the way as the pregnancy progresses, but in one in 10 cases it remains in this position[55]. The position of your placenta is noted at your 20-week scan and, if it appears low, you will be offered another scan at around 32 weeks to reassess it. Often those with a placenta praevia will need to have a C-section to deliver their baby, as the placenta is blocking the birthing canal.

Placental abruption – this occurs when the placenta separates from the inside wall of the womb before birth. It affects up to one in 100 pregnancies[56], and its complication rate can depend on the severity of the abruption and how far along in your pregnancy you are.

Vasa praevia – a very rare condition affecting between one in 1,200 and one in 5,000 pregnancies[57] and occurs when the blood vessels connecting your baby to your placenta run close to the cervix. These vessels are delicate and are at risk of tearing, which can be dangerous for the baby. This, however, is most likely to occur when your waters break, so you would be offered a preterm C-section.

WHAT SHOULD YOU DO IF YOU ARE BLEEDING?

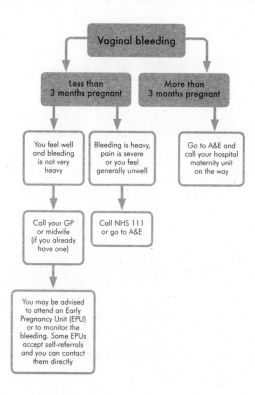

REDUCED FOETAL MOVEMENTS

Most women are aware of their baby moving by 20 weeks, though if your placenta is at the front of your womb, it can be more difficult to feel your baby's movements. The number of movements tends to increase until 32 weeks, then plateau until labour. Your baby will sleep throughout the day and night, and there may be periods between 20 and 40 minutes that you do not notice your baby moving. However, if you notice your baby moving less than normal, it can be a sign of distress, and you will need to be assessed. If you are unsure whether movements are reduced after 28 weeks of gestation, try lying on your left side and focus on foetal movements for 2 hours. If you do not feel ten or more discrete movements in 2 hours, you should contact your midwife or maternity unit immediately.

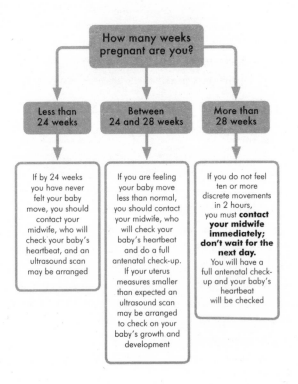

GROUP B STREPTOCOCCUS (GBS)

Group B Streptococcus (GBS) is a bacteria naturally found in our digestive, genital and urinary tracts. It can spread from person to person through contact with bodily fluids like respiratory secretions, urine and faeces. If a pregnant woman carries the bacteria, it can also be transmitted to the newborn during childbirth.

Around 20–40 per cent of pregnant women carry GBS with no symptoms[58]. Whilst it is usually harmless to healthy adults and considered a regular part of our flora, in some rare cases it can pose a risk to newborns, with some even suffering from severe and life-threatening infections like sepsis, pneumonia and meningitis. GBS accounts for around a third of neonatal sepsis cases[59].

As such, some countries screen for GBS in pregnant women with a vaginal/rectal swab between 35 and 37 weeks of pregnancy. If it is detected, the mother is given intravenous antibiotics during labour to reduce the risk of it being transmitted to the baby. In the UK, however, we do not routinely screen for GBS, though it can be incidentally picked up on a urine test or a vaginal or rectal swab that is done for other purposes. It is not routinely screened for in the UK primarily due to the ratio of risks to benefits.

Without treatment, around 50 per cent of mothers pass the GBS onto their babies, but only approximately 1 per cent end up with a clinical infection[60]. This equates to around one in 1,000 babies with a clinical infection (around 20 per cent of the population × 50 per cent transmission rate × 1 per cent clinically infected). In the UK, it is estimated that 440 mothers would need to receive antibiotics to prevent one case of disease and 3,000 to prevent one case leading to death or severe disability[61]. This very large number of women that need to be unnecessarily treated with antibiotics to prevent a single case of neonatal sepsis, together with the risks associated with antibiotics (for example, consider the microbiome) and antibiotic resistance, makes for a case against screening for GBS.

Furthermore, when we compare our results to the US, which does screen for GBS, the incidence of disease as a result of GBS is currently comparable[62]. This suggests that screening for GBS means that thousands of women are being given antibiotics with little evidence to suggest it helps to reduce mortality from the disease.

If you choose to take the GBS test privately and it is positive, or you are incidentally found to have GBS, there are a few measures that might be taken. You may be advised to review your birthing plan to ensure you are having your baby in the hospital, and to contact your midwife as soon as your waters break or you go into labour. In addition to the antibiotics you will be given during labour, you may also be advised to stay in hospital for at least 12 hours postnatally.

PREGNANCY: A TIRED MAMMA'S SUMMARY

Forbidden foods: some foods should be avoided during pregnancy due to possible bacterial contamination or potential harm to the foetus, including certain cheeses, fish, meats, eggs and caffeine.

Weight in pregnancy: weight gain during pregnancy is a natural and necessary process involving various components beyond body fat. The importance of balanced nutrition and mindful weight management should come above any dieting.

Exercise in pregnancy: the benefits of exercising during pregnancy include maintaining cardiovascular fitness, managing weight, reducing the risk of complications and improving mood. Consideration should be made for activities like contact sports, overheating and heavy weights, due to pregnancy-related changes.

Sleep issues: hormonal changes, congestion, reflux, discomfort and anxiety can contribute to sleep disturbances. The recommendation to sleep on your side from the third trimester onwards reduces the risk of stillbirth.

Prenatal scans: the 12-week scan (dating scan) and the 20-week scan (anomaly scan) offer insights into the baby's development, estimated due date and potential health issues. The nuchal translucency measurement, part of the combined test, assesses the risk of Down's syndrome, Edwards' syndrome and Patau's syndrome. Alongside the scans you will also be offered various antenatal screening tests, including blood tests for conditions like thalassaemia, sickle cell disease, HIV, hepatitis B and syphilis.

Vaccinations: the following vaccinations are currently recommended to protect the pregnant person and the developing baby: flu, whooping cough and Covid-19.

Glucose tolerance test (GTT): GTT assesses how well the body processes sugar and is used to diagnose gestational diabetes mellitus (GDM). GDM can lead to various pregnancy complications. Factors like age, BMI, previous gestational diabetes, family history and ethnicity can increase the risk of GDM. The GTT procedure involves fasting overnight, having a blood test, consuming a glucose drink and having a follow-up blood test.

PREGNANCY COMPLICATIONS:

Deep vein thrombosis (DVT): pregnancy increases the risk of DVT, especially after birth. Heparin injections are used to treat DVT, and epidurals may be delayed if injections are ongoing.

High blood pressure: gestational hypertension and pre-eclampsia can develop during pregnancy, affecting blood pressure and potentially leading to complications for both the pregnant person and the baby. Monitoring and medication may be necessary.

Intrahepatic cholestasis: this liver condition can cause itching and other issues. It can lead to complications for the baby and may require earlier delivery.

Hyperemesis gravidarum: severe nausea and vomiting can lead to dehydration and weight loss. Treatment includes fluids, medication and monitoring.

Unexpected bleeding: bleeding during pregnancy can have various causes, including implantation, cervical changes, infection, or more serious conditions like placental abruption. Not all bleeding indicates a miscarriage.

Group B Streptococcus (GBS): GBS is a bacteria that can be transmitted to the baby during childbirth. Some countries screen for GBS, while others, like the UK, do not routinely screen, due to the ratio of risks to benefits. Antibiotics may be given to reduce the risk of transmission.

CHAPTER 4

PREPARING FOR LABOUR

BE PREPARED

BIRTH PLANS

From the moment that pregnancy test flashes up as positive, you have an endless stream of decisions to make about the birth. I know some people who have taken the 'bury your head in the sand' approach and just hope the decisions will be made for them. Others have taken a more 'come what may' approach and made decisions as they faced them. Then you have people like me, who feel that doing the research and being as well informed as possible before will allow for the best decision making. I suspect if you are reading this book in preparation for your upcoming parenthood, you are already most likely to be this latter person.

Your midwife will encourage you to formulate a birth plan, a document stating what you would like to happen during labour and after birth. This ensures that you have thought about the most likely eventualities, where relevant, that you have discussed things with your partner, and that your midwife understands your priorities. In every decision made, you need to consider the options and also question the risks and benefits of these to you and your baby. Your pregnancy notes given to you by the midwife may have a template to follow, though the questions needing answering are as follows. These do not need to be binary yes or no answers, but rather you can state preferences if that sits better with you. Remember, it is ok to say you don't know yet, and just because it is written in a birth plan, it is by no means finite. You can change your mind, and sometimes circumstances will change it for you. In fact, many now refer to it as a birth 'guide', to relieve the pressure and anxiety should your birth not go to 'plan'.

- Where do you intend to give birth? If you can, be specific about the environment and why you have chosen this place, but if you aren't sure, detail the feeling you would like to achieve. Would you like music, diffusers and dark lighting? Would you be happy for students to be present?
- Would you like a birthing partner? Many people choose to have a birthing partner(s) with them. Detail what you would and wouldn't like your birthing partner to do. Do you still want them there if you have a forceps/ventouse delivery or need a C-section?
- Do you want any special equipment? Would you like to use a birthing ball, bean bags or mats?
- Do you want to use a birthing pool or any other special facility?
- How do you feel about monitoring during labour? Consider whether you would be happy to have regular vaginal examinations to monitor your progress throughout labour and what kind of monitoring you would like for the baby's heartbeat (continual sonar foetal monitoring or hand-held Doppler/stethoscope).
- What position would you like to be in for birth? Consider whether you want to squat, sit, kneel, lie down or stand.
- What pain relief would you like? Would you like to be offered pain relief and, if so, are you open to a TENS machine (see page 123), gas and air, pethidine, an epidural or spinal block?
- Would you like immediate skin-to-skin contact? Your baby can be passed to you as soon as you give birth and placed on your chest for skin-to-skin contact. Or your baby can be cleaned and wrapped in a blanket first.
- Would you like your partner to receive the baby or announce the sex?
- Would you like a delayed cord cutting? Would you like your partner to cut the cord?
- What are your feelings about an episiotomy? If the perineum (the space between the vagina and anus) does not stretch enough, it can be

at risk of tearing, and an episiotomy (a cut between these two areas) can be considered to reduce the risk of tearing or to help deliver the baby quickly if there are any concerns.

- How would you like your placenta delivered? You can consider a natural delivery or a managed placental delivery, where an injection is given to help the womb contract. Would you like to keep your placenta?
- Are you happy for your baby to have vitamin K and, if so, how would you like it administered? Vitamin K helps your baby form blood clots, it can be administered orally or by injection.
- How would you like to feed your baby? You can consider breastfeeding, bottle feeding, or a mixture of both. Would you like support in establishing breastfeeding?
- Have you any other special requests? Have you been practising hypnobirthing, and would you like support to ensure that you are able to practise it throughout? Do you have any religious requirements? Do you need an interpreter? Do you have special dietary needs? Do you or your partner have any special needs?

For my birth plan, I followed the standard template in my maternity notes, but you should feel free to get creative. You might prefer more visual aids to depict your preferences, or find your brain works better with mind-mapping your thoughts onto paper.

I once read an article about the birthing rituals of the Huichol people, an indigenous Mexican tribe. The piece claimed that the father would sit above the labouring wife in the rafters of the hut with a rope tied around his testicles, and when the labouring woman felt a painful contraction, she would pull on the rope so that he, too, would experience the pain of childbirth. Whether or not this folklore was true, I seriously considered adding it to my birth plan.

WHERE TO GIVE BIRTH

There are a few options available to expectant parents when it comes to choosing where to give birth, from traditional hospital births to more intimate home births. The decision of where to give birth is a deeply personal one, and it may be determined by cultural influences, your medical history, your support system or simply individual preferences. By understanding the features of each potential birth space, it is easier to have the confidence to choose the environment that aligns with your own values and aspirations.

LABOUR WARD

As a doctor, I am naturally risk averse, and having seen first-hand the possible complications of labour, I always thought I would give birth in a labour ward. It's a bit like opting for a Sunday roast with all the trimmings – I wanted obstetricians, midwives, paediatricians, forceps, drugs; all the interventions.

The labour ward, sometimes known as the delivery suite, is located within the hospital and has doctors on hand if needed, with all the medical equipment. Some labour wards also have birthing pools, balls and other equipment available, though it is unlikely that every room will have these, so you may not have this as an option. You will have your own room for the labour, though you may have to stay on a communal, less-private ward postnatally. You also have a wide range of pain relief available to you, including epidurals, should you decide you want it. This tends to be an ideal option for women who have medical conditions or complications of pregnancy and are at higher risk of requiring medical interventions.

BIRTHING CENTRE

Suddenly, on falling pregnant, the woo-woo Mother Earth in me just took over! I hadn't entirely succumbed to wanting a home birth, but I was keen on having a more homely environment to welcome my newborn into and was really keen on water birth. A birth centre can be located at the hospital, alongside a labour ward, or in a separate unit or building. They are more likely to have birthing pools available and other equipment to help coach you through your labour. As they are midwife-run, they are not set up to offer epidurals but are more experienced in natural pain relief methods.

HOME BIRTH

During my pregnancy, Covid struck, and the rules about partners being present during labour changed, so I did a 180 and opted for a home birth. I remember telling a friend of mine, who is a paediatrician, my plans and watching his face drop. He told me every horror story he had heard to try to get me to change my mind. I understood his concern, we know that 45 per cent of women who were planning to have their first baby at home end up being transferred to a hospital while in labour or just after birth[63]. To compound that, ambulances were already at their capacity with Covid patients, and he worried that if I needed to be transferred as an emergency, there wouldn't be an ambulance available. Despite having never been pregnant or having any precedent, somehow, for me, I knew that being in a comfortable environment, with my husband and my own bed, was what I needed for my labour to progress without complication. Home births offer familiarity, the option to have as many people as you want there with you, the guarantee of a birthing pool, if that's what you want, and having a midwife all to yourself. (I know this might sound like a luxury, but all NHS Trusts are expected to run a home birth service, though it is not guaranteed by law. If the Trust has shortages, they have an obligation to provide staff for the service they offer, even if that means outsourcing to independent midwives. So, you shouldn't be in a situation to have a home birth denied due to staff numbers.) While pain relief options are more limited, your midwife can still bring gas and air. The other possible downside is that you have to prep everything, so you need to ensure the birthing pool is set up, and you must have all the towels and sheets you will need, clean and ready.

ANTENATAL CLASSES

Antenatal classes are optional but can be helpful, especially if it is your first pregnancy. They start from around 30–32 weeks of pregnancy and are designed to help you navigate through the confusing world of pregnancy, labour and early parenthood. They are also a good way to meet people who will be on maternity leave at the same time as you (see page 175, Find your crew). You can attend free local NHS classes, or you can opt to pay for one of the many private groups. Either way, they get filled up early, so book your place as soon as you feel comfortable doing so.

Whilst the classes can vary depending on area, in general, here is the low-down for NHS vs private antenatal classes:

	NHS	Private
Number of classes	Usually around 2 hours. They can vary between one class and several weekly classes.	10–20 hours over several weeks.
Where do they take place?	They often take place in hospitals.	They can be in pubs, halls, social clubs – pretty much anywhere.
Who runs the class?	Usually midwives.	Usually, midwives or people qualified as antenatal teachers.
Cost	Free.	Varies around the country, on average £200–500.
Class size	Variable.	Varies between 2 and 15 couples.
Who can attend?	Some classes are just for you, others your partner can attend.	Most welcome partners, but not all of them.

I opted for the private classes for two reasons. Firstly, they were in the evenings, which meant I could still attend without having to miss any work; and, secondly, because the one I chose was set in a pub and I thought that bribing my husband with Pale Ale was the best way to keep him engaged! However, Covid then hit, and the rest of the course took place via Zoom, from our sofa, with cups of tea and he was pretty disappointed.

HYPNOBIRTHING

Hypnobirthing was such an incredible process for me that I have to shout about it now. I know it sounds very hemp-wearing and tree-hugging, but, honestly, it doesn't have to be any of those things (unless, of course, that is your jam) – it is actually very logical and is based on the physiology of our bodies. I knew about hypnobirthing peripherally and had started listening to some audiobooks during early pregnancy, but I really submerged myself in it after covering the topic on *This Morning*, after the Princess of Wales had revealed on a podcast that she found it hugely helpful. She said, *'I saw the power of it, the meditation and the deep breathing and things like that, that they teach you in hypno-birthing when I was really sick. I'm not going to say that William was standing there chanting sweet nothings at me. He definitely wasn't! It had been so bad during pregnancy, I actually really quite liked labour.'*

Hypnobirthing is a way to prepare yourself for childbirth that emphasises relaxation, self-hypnosis and visualisation techniques to help you achieve a calm and comfortable birth experience. The philosophy is based on the work of British obstetrician Mr Grantly Dick-Read, who believed that fear and tension were the main causes of pain during childbirth (I think he may have omitted to consider the watermelon-sized object being ejected through your vagina, but I do agree that fear adds to pain). Hypnobirthing can be beneficial not just for mothers but also for their birth partners, who can learn techniques to help support them during labour.

Hypnobirthing reduces anxiety, fear and pain during childbirth by teaching women to trust their bodies and work with the natural birthing process. I have nothing to compare it to as I have only had one birth, but I genuinely felt empowered during labour. Sometimes I felt out of control, but there was no time that I doubted my body could do this.

Hypnobirthing classes typically teach deep-breathing exercises, visualisation techniques and positive affirmations to promote relaxation and reduce stress. They may also include education about the physiology of childbirth, pain management techniques and the different stages of labour. I didn't attend any hypnobirthing classes, but I read books and listened to audiobooks, which worked well for me and my schedule (and was also convenient during lockdown).

The practice of hypnobirthing is based on the belief that childbirth does not have to be a traumatic or painful experience and that you can create a positive and empowering birth experience for you and your baby. A birth free from medical interventions cannot be guaranteed, nor is hypnobirthing meant to replace medical intervention, but some choose to use the methods as an alternative to pain relief, or in conjunction with medical interventions like epidurals, Caesarean sections or induction.

There are five standard hypnobirthing techniques:

Relaxation techniques – hypnobirthing emphasises relaxation as a critical aspect of managing pain during labour. Deep breathing, progressive muscle relaxation and visualisation can help women stay calm and focused during childbirth.

Affirmations – positive affirmations are used to help women feel confident and empowered during labour. These affirmations may be written or spoken and can help women feel more in control of the birthing process. I had affirmations written out on revision cue cards and stuck all over my house. I couldn't take a poo without reading things like 'I embrace the power of birth', and 'All is calm, all is well, I am safe'!

Self-hypnosis – hypnobirthing often involves techniques to help women reach a state of deep relaxation and focus during labour, helping them manage pain and reduce anxiety. This is not a technique I learnt in my readings, but it is likely something you would learn if you attended the classes.

Birth rehearsal imagery – this technique involves mentally rehearsing the birth process beforehand, visualising a positive and comfortable birth experience, and helping women feel more prepared and confident when the time comes.

Massage – gentle touch and massage can help to release tension and promote relaxation during labour. Partners or doulas may use massage techniques to support the labouring woman.

Lesser-known hypnobirthing techniques include 'fear release', which involves identifying and releasing any fears or negative beliefs around childbirth that may hinder the birthing process, and birth partner hypnosis, which involves teaching the birth partner self-hypnosis techniques to help them remain calm and supportive during labour.

There are many reports out there suggesting hypnobirthing is the panacea to manage pain, reduce anxiety and have a more positive birth experience. The quality of some of these studies is dubious. However, one trusted Cochrane Review found that fewer women who did hypnobirthing needed pain relief for labour (although the rates of epidurals were the same)[64]. Another systematic review and meta-analysis of 10 studies found that hypnobirthing was associated with reduced fear of childbirth and a lower likelihood of needing medical interventions[65]. And another 2015 study found that women generally appreciated hypnobirthing training and found it beneficial[66]. Based on this research, the Royal College of Midwives and the National Institute for Health and Care Excellence[67] have both endorsed hypnobirthing as a safe and effective way to manage pain and anxiety during labour and to promote a positive birth experience.

While there is no one-size-fits-all approach to childbirth, hypnobirthing may be a helpful tool for many women to manage pain, reduce anxiety and have a more positive birth experience.

COLOSTRUM HARVESTING

Early breast milk is perfectly tailored to your new baby's immunological and nutritional needs. We start producing it well before the baby arrives, as early as 16 weeks. This early breast milk is known as colostrum. It is yellow, sticky, thick and often called 'liquid gold', and it can be hand-expressed and harvested from 36 weeks of pregnancy, ready for your baby after birth, should they need it. It is a concentrated liquid, which is necessary because your newborn baby's stomach is only tiny (the size of a marble) and is only able to take in small amounts. It contains higher amounts of protein, and less fat and sugar, which is easier for a newborn to digest.

As well as being high in nutrition, colostrum contains the antibodies needed to help your baby's immune system defend them against infections. It protects them from allergies by helping their digestive system and microbiome develop. Finally, it reduces your baby's risk of jaundice by acting as a laxative and encouraging their bowels to open and pass the first black, sticky poo known as meconium. Research has also shown that women that hand-express in pregnancy are more confident and better prepared to breastfeed their babies.[68]

Harvesting the colostrum is essentially a backup plan in case your baby is unable to breastfeed initially or has any challenges in doing so. Those that may benefit the most from colostrum harvesting are babies that have issues with maintaining their blood sugar levels. This can occur if your baby is large or small for their gestational age, or if they are diagnosed with a cleft lip and/or palate or other congenital conditions. It might also be beneficial to harvest colostrum if you have diabetes or have gestational diabetes, you are taking a beta blocker for raised blood pressure, you are electing for a Caesarean birth, or you have had previous breast surgery. There may be other conditions, and your midwife can advise whether or not you should consider harvesting colostrum.

Some women, including those at risk of preterm labour, have a history of preterm ruptured membranes (when your waters break early), or if you have a cervical suture, should NOT harvest colostrum. This is because of the risk that hand-expressing can bring on contractions, which is why you are not advised to do it before 36 weeks of pregnancy.

HOW TO COLLECT COLOSTRUM

To collect the colostrum, you only need a 1ml syringe – although some people prefer to collect it into a sterilised cup first and then suck it up into the syringe – and some labels.

1. Find a time when you are relaxed and are not feeling rushed, then get your equipment ready and wash your hands.
2. Cup one breast with one hand, then with the other hand, hold it around 2–3cm back from your nipple (just outside the darker area called the areola) in a C-shape with your thumb and the rest of your fingers, and gently squeeze.
3. Release the pressure, then repeat again and again until you have a rhythm going. The first time you do this, you may only get a few drops (if anything) but as you build your supply, you will get more. Suck up the drops into the syringe, or if that is too tricky to coordinate, scoop it into the cup.
4. When the flow slows down, move your hand around to cup a different section of your breast, then repeat.
5. If the flow stops or slows, move to the other breast and repeat the same action.
6. Label each syringe with your name, hospital number and date of birth, and the date and time the colostrum was expressed.

You can store it in the fridge at a temperature of 2–4°C and add to it for up to 48 hours, but after 48 hours you should place the syringe(s) in a clean ziplock bag and store the colostrum in your freezer at a temperature of –18°C. When the time comes to go to the hospital, the frozen colostrum can be transported with you in a cool bag to keep it as frozen as possible. Once thawed, it must be used within 24 hours, but it should be kept chilled at all times. Colostrum harvesting should be done for no more than 3–5 minutes at one time, two to three times a day.

Don't worry if you can't get much out when you try; it does not reflect your breastfeeding journey. I only managed to express a tiny amount, which stressed me more than it should have, but once Harris came, milk supply was never an issue for me.

Some tips that may help you get more flow can include gently massaging the breasts before you start and readjusting the distance from your nipple to closer or further away (but try to avoid pressing on the nipple itself as this may become sore). This method of hand-expressing the colostrum is also how you could hand-express milk once the baby arrives, so, even if the colostrum harvesting hasn't been as fruitful as you would like, you have still learnt a skill that may be useful later.

PERINEAL MASSAGE

I'm putting it out there; I hated doing this. I found it uncomfortable and awkward with my massive bump, and I found any excuse not to have to do it. But then I suffered with tears during birth, so do as I say and not as I do!

Perineal massage is the process of gradually softening and stretching the perineum to prepare it for birth. The perineum is the area of skin between the vagina and anus which naturally stretches to allow for the passage of your baby during birth, but it can sometimes result in tears. An estimated 85 per cent of women who have vaginal births will tear, with around two-thirds requiring stitches[69].

However, studies have shown that regular perineal massage from 35 weeks of pregnancy can reduce the risk of tears needing stitches by 10 per cent or needing an episiotomy (see page 112) by 16 per cent in first-time mothers[70]. Studies have also shown that in women who have given birth before, perineal massage was reported to reduce the ongoing perineal pain by 32 per cent at three months postpartum[71], though it did not improve sexual satisfaction or pain on sexual intercourse 3 months after giving birth. Interestingly, there seems to be no risk reduction in those with first-degree tears (minor abrasions to the skin which don't need stitches), or third- and fourth-degree tears, which are more complicated injuries to the anal sphincter muscle. It also did not reduce the need for an assisted delivery with forceps or ventouse, making no difference to bladder or bowel functioning after birth.

Using a warm compress on your perineum during the second stage of labour (pushing) may also help reduce the risk of perineal tears.

HOW TO DO PERINEAL MASSAGE

Preparation

1. You will need to wash your hands and cut your nails. Longer nails will feel uncomfortable and irritating, and can damage your perineum's delicate skin and tissue.
2. Choose an unscented lubricant. This can be a personal lubricant like KY Jelly or a natural oil like olive or almond oil. You can even buy oils that are specifically marketed for perineal massage.
3. Get a mirror so you can see what you are doing.
4. Find a comfortable position. Most people will sit up propped by some pillows on their sofa or bed, but, truly, just find what works for you – whether in a bath, shower or on the loo. It can be easier if you have a warm bath first, as it can make the tissues feel softer to massage.

Doing the deed

1. Put some lubricant on the lower part of your vaginal opening and relax.
2. Put your thumbs around 2.5–4cm inside your vagina.
3. Press your thumbs down towards the back passage, hold them there for 1–2 minutes, then move the thumbs in an upwards and outwards, U-shaped movement.
4. Repeat this a few times. You will feel a stretching or pressure sensation, though it should not hurt, and you should stop if it does.

Aim for 5–10 minutes a day, or longer if you're loving it!

You can also involve your partner, who can help you with the massage, especially in the latter weeks when you feel like a huge whale and can barely reach your vagina, let alone massage it. It might be easier for your partner to use their index fingers rather than thumbs.

PELVIC FLOOR EXERCISES

We should all be doing pelvic floor exercises – always, not just during pregnancy. Your pelvic floor muscles are put under more pressure due to the growing weight of your baby, as well as being impacted by hormonal changes, which means that your pelvic floor needs extra TLC during pregnancy.

Your pelvic floor comprises layers of muscles that act like a sling, attaching at the back to the tailbone (coccyx) and the front at the pubic bone, supporting the weight of the pelvic organs, which are the bladder, bowels and womb. When the pelvic floor muscles are not functioning optimally, you may develop incontinence of urine when you cough, sneeze, laugh and jump, develop an urgency of passing urine, leak stool from your back passage, or find sex painful or not as pleasurable.

Over a third of women experience urinary incontinence in the second and third trimesters, and a third continue to experience this in the first three months postpartum[72]. However, just like any other muscle, the pelvic floor muscles can be strengthened through regular exercise to help avoid this. In addition to helping to prevent incontinence, pelvic floor exercises have also been found to help you ease your baby out during labour and recover faster after birth.

Here goes a moment of TMI – I never experienced urinary incontinence, but I rolled over in bed in my final trimester and sharted. That was enough of a reminder to me, until my dying days, to do my pelvic floor exercises. I never again want to scoop my own poop from my knickers.

HOW TO DO PELVIC FLOOR EXERCISES

The beauty of pelvic floor exercises is that they can be done practically anywhere. They involve trying to squeeze and lift the pelvic floor by tightening up your back passage (not clenching your buttocks), as if you're trying your hardest not to fart in front of your very proper mother-in-law, then think about lifting upwards and forwards to your pubic bone. After every squeeze make sure you fully relax the muscles as well. You want to avoid holding your breath when you do them, so practise breathing out as your squeeze and breathing in as you relax. There are two types of pelvic floor exercises to do: the short squeeze and the long squeeze.

The short squeeze

1. Squeeze your pelvic floor muscles, then hold for 1 second.
2. Relax fully.
3. Repeat up to 10 times.

The long squeeze

1. Squeeze your pelvic floor, then hold it for 10 seconds. You may not be able to do 10 seconds to start with. Try 4 seconds (or less if needed) and gradually increase the hold length as you practise. Remember to breathe normally whilst you hold, don't hold your breath.
2. Release and relax fully for 4 seconds.
3. Repeat up to 10 times.

The aim is to do an equal mixture of quick and slow squeezes around three times daily. Perhaps it can be your mealtime ritual, getting the whole family involved! There are also several apps available to remind you and guide you through the exercises, and many new gadgets and devices on the market. I thoroughly recommend the apps, as their insistent reminders make it hard for you to ignore (I used the NHS Squeezy app), but the gadgets are not necessary for all and some are not suitable for use in pregnancy, but can be used in the postnatal period.

Clare Bourne, a pelvic health physiotherapist, discusses the devices on the market:

'There are two main types of devices: stimulation devices and biofeedback devices. Stimulation devices include a probe placed inside the vagina, connected to a handheld device, which activates the pelvic floor for you. These are good for those who cannot contract their pelvic floor themselves, however, they are not appropriate for use in pregnancy. Biofeedback devices also include an internal probe and connect to a handheld device with wires or via Bluetooth. These can help to give you visual feedback of what your pelvic floor is able to do, and help to motivate you as you do them. Many brands can be used in pregnancy, but some only in the second and third trimesters. Always check the instruction manual of the device before.'

As with most exercises, it is easy to find excuses not to do them, but, in most cases, pelvic floor exercises can be done sitting at your desk, in a traffic jam, while watching TV or eating dinner. So it's time to flex those multitasking and pelvic muscles.

HOSPITAL 'GRAB' BAG CHECKLIST

Although I ended up having a home birth and thankfully didn't need to transfer to the hospital during or after the birth, I still packed a hospital bag to grab and go just in case. The possibilities of what you can pack seem endless; I'm sure there were things I had forgotten, but here is my checklist, copied and pasted straight out of my iPhone notes! I've added some extra notes to some of them, so you know what I found most useful and what I didn't.

For Mama

Item	Comments
Hospital notes	They go everywhere with you.
Hypnobirthing book	This was a bit of a bible for me, it went everywhere with me (see section about hypnobirthing).
PJs – front-opening top and nightie	I had bought this amazingly soft and wonderful nightdress especially for after birth, as I wanted to feel as comfy and luxurious as possible. I was so excited to wear it. Turns out my boobs got big and it just didn't fit properly anymore. So just think practical, baggy and washable! A nightie is more comfortable if you have a C-section, as the waistband won't rub.
Phone charger	Obvious.

Item	Comments
Snacks and drinks	My gorgeous friends made me a hamper of scrumptious snacks for my baby shower – such a thoughtful and helpful gift. I remember eating my way through all the snacks in bed with my bub in my arms. Perfection.
The pillow	I find that hospital laundry has a certain smell to it, and the cotton is pretty industrial and rough, so I wanted to have my own fluffy pillow and soft pillowcase.
TENS machine	I used the hell out of mine at the initial stages of labour. I have no idea if it helped, but I think, if anything, it offered a distraction and something for me to do.
Toothbrush and toothpaste	
Deodorant	
Hairbrush/tangle tease	
Face wipes	
Moisturiser	
Towel	Hospital towels feel like sandpaper.
Birthing ball	They are likely to have these in the birthing centres, but they may not have enough if it's a busy day.
Maternity pads	There is nothing elegant about these pads. You feel like an infant wearing a nappy. But they are big and stop you from leaking all over the shop.
Granny pants	Get the biggest, most comfy cotton pants you can find. In case of a C-section, you want a cut that will not rub against the scar, so think high-waisted rather than some sexy Brazilian brief.

Item	Comments
Disposable pants	When there are lots of fluids coming out of you from various orifices, tears and incisions, the best thing you can do is chuck away your pants and start again!
Dressing gown	
Flip-flops	
Socks	
Comfy outfit to wear home	Make sure it has a loose waistband in case of a C-section.
Cash	I know that nowadays everything can be paid for by card/phone, but somewhere in the back of my head is a parental figure saying, 'Always have cash on you, just in case.'
iPad	Download your happy films and videos, ready for when you need a little pick-me-up.
Headphones or ear plugs	Having spent a significant period of my medical training in hospitals, taking a history from a patient behind one curtain, only to hear the straining noises followed by plops and a sigh behind the adjacent curtain, I knew the absolute necessity of headphones. Preferably noise-cancelling ones!
Nursing bras	When your milk comes in, your boobs become two angry watermelons and you will be grateful for the support of your nursing bras. They're so comfy, and two years on I still wear them, so invest in some good ones. You'll want to wear them forever!
Breast pads	For those leaky titty moments.
Water bottle with a straw	Pretend you're sipping a cocktail from a flamingo straw on a beach somewhere, not in Colchester, having your vagina prised open.

Item	Comments
Peri bottle	Best purchase of 2020! Given how much I rave about how important this is, I should invest in shares. On giving birth, you may have tears and even the superficial ones, when in contact with your acidic urine, burn like Hades. So by squeezing water at your vulva as you pass urine, you are diluting the urine, making it far less irritant.
Dry shampoo	Because not everyone can come out of labour with a Kate Middleton blow dry.
Bikini and a big T-shirt	I wasn't sure how 'shy' I would feel having to sit in a birthing pool naked in front of strangers, so I packed these in case a bit of self-consciousness came over me.
Rupert's swim shorts	He definitely didn't need to be naked!
Positive affirmations	I had written these on cue cards to stick up around me during labour.
Hot water bottle	If it works for period cramps, surely it'll work for labour! Right??!
Fan	So you can look like you're in a Beyoncé music video whilst keeping cool.
Eye mask	Fluorescent-lit hospitals play havoc with your circadian rhythm and melatonin levels.
Speakers	To play the hell out of those power ballads you have put on your labour playlist.
Diffuser and lavender oil	So you can pretend you are actually at a Cowshed Spa having a facial.
Lip balm	Because all that screaming at your birthing partner makes for cracked lips.

Item	Comments
Sieve for the birthing pool	I didn't even poo myself (hurrah!), so that sieve ended up being used for cooking at home – no waste in the Kayat kitchen!
Hair ties	My hair has a life of its own and after 9 months of no shedding, it needed securing in about 15 different ways.
Lanolin	Your nipples' best friend.

For Baby

Item	Comments
Baby vests x2	I packed two sizes, newborn and tiny.
Baby sleepsuit x2	Again, I packed two sizes, but also I cannot tell you how much getting the ones that zip up rather than the ones that snap will help your sanity. When you're exhausted and on the 100th outfit change of the day, trying to make the snaps line up will feel like trying to solve a Rubik's cube. Zips are an easy solution to that.
Hat	
Scratch mittens	
Socks	
Nappies	
Wet wipes	
Cotton wool pads	The cold temperatures of wet wipes would just startle and upset Harris, so we used cotton wool pads and warm water to clean him for at least the first month. It also felt much kinder for his very delicate newborn skin.

Item	Comments
Cellular cotton blanket	
Muslin squares	
Sterilised bottles	
Formula	I intended to breastfeed, but I also didn't want to be in a situation where I wasn't able to, and I felt trapped. So I took some 'just in case' formula.
Frozen colostrum	See the section on colostrum harvesting.
Car seat	This is a prerequisite to being discharged, so do not forget it.

DUE DATES

Both the medical profession and pregnant women tend to follow due dates as if they are an exact science, but, actually, only 5 per cent of births arrive on their due date[73]. It implies that all babies are ready to be born after the same time of pregnancy, but we know that babies often reach milestones at different times, so the same can be considered with time in the womb. However, it is a 'normal' full-term pregnancy if you deliver any time between 37 and 42 weeks of pregnancy. That's a whole 5 weeks of variation!

The estimated due date (EDD) is calculated by counting 280 days from the first day of your last period. This calculation is based on the presumption that you do not know your exact conception date, but, if you do, it can be calculated as 266 days from that date. When you calculate the EDD from the first date of your last period, it makes the assumption that you have a 28-day cycle and that you ovulated on day 14. However, we know that there is a lot of variation on cycle length and ovulation date, and we also know that the time between conception and fertilisation, and the time between fertilisation and implantation, can vary too. These variations can all result in inaccuracies in calculating the EDD in this way. This is why the EDD is further refined by estimating your baby's size from measurements during the ultrasound scan. Still, it is not perfect, and a study using women who conceived by IVF and therefore knew the exact date their egg was fertilised found that the ultrasound dating scan often estimated an earlier due date by an average of 3 days[74].

So, given a term pregnancy can be within a significant range and the EDD is not always accurate, you might ask why the EDD actually matters. It is primarily useful as a tool to help us plot your baby's development and growth through the pregnancy. However, it is also a marker of when a baby's delivery might be premature (<37 weeks) or overdue (>42 weeks) and what this could mean for you and them. Born too early and the baby may not be fully prepared for life outside of the cosy womb, and may need special assistance, born too late and there may be increased complications associated with longer pregnancies, like larger birth weight and high blood pressure. Induction of labour is usually offered by 42 weeks of pregnancy to avoid these complications, and sometimes earlier in certain circumstances.

Table showing the percentage of when each labour usually occurs[75]

Week of pregnancy	Percentage of recorded births
41 weeks or later	6.5
39–41	57.5
37–38	26
34–36	7
Before 34	3

PREPARING FOR LABOUR: A TIRED MAMMA'S SUMMARY

Birth plan: the questions and considerations to be addressed in a birth plan include the choice of birth environment, birthing partner preferences, special equipment, pain relief options, birthing positions, immediate skin-to-skin contact, cord cutting, placenta delivery, vitamin K administration, feeding choices and other special requests.

Antenatal classes: these are optional but can provide valuable information and support for first-time parents.

Hypnobirthing: a technique that promotes relaxation, self-hypnosis and visualisation to manage pain and anxiety during childbirth.

Colostrum harvesting: the process of collecting early breast milk can provide nutrition and immune support to newborns. Start from 36 weeks pregnant.

Perineal massage: a technique to prepare the perineum for birth and reduce the risk of tears during delivery. Start from 35 weeks pregnant.

Pelvic floor exercises: exercises to prevent issues like incontinence and to aid in labour and recovery. You can do these leading up to, during and after pregnancy.

Due dates: the calculation of estimated due dates (EDDs) is primarily a tool for tracking foetal development and growth. Term pregnancy can occur between 37 and 42 weeks.

Bringing on labour naturally: a number of methods have been documented, including walking, consuming dates, raspberry leaf tea, sex, spicy food, acupuncture, pineapples and nipple stimulation. Though the effectiveness of all of these have not been proven.

Induced labour: a medical procedure to artificially bring about childbirth when labour doesn't start on its own or when there are medical reasons to expedite the process. Common reasons for induction include reaching 41 weeks of pregnancy, medical issues and potential risks for the baby. The process of labour induction can include the use of a 'sweep' to stimulate labour, the insertion of a catheter balloon to soften the cervix, administration of prostaglandin gels or tablets, artificial rupture of membranes, and the use of synthetic oxytocin via intravenous drip.

CHAPTER 5

LABOUR BE PREPARED

It seems so common to hear about traumatic birth stories – the one where a friend is left in a hospital bed in a corridor for hours, the cousin who had a 72-hour labour, the mum who was ripped from front to back, the emergency C-sections and the pain. But mine was lovely and simple, and I thought I'd share it here with you.

MY BIRTH STORY

It was 10 May, and I was recording a podcast, during which I started getting some pain in my lower abdomen. We joked on the podcast that I was going into labour, but it was a fleeting comment, as I wasn't due until 23 May, and everyone 'knows' that your first baby is always late, right? I went for a wee and the pain went away, so I ignored it, but in retrospect this was probably the beginning.

In the following couple of days I did quite a few online yoga and fitness classes to make sure I was fit for labour. Honestly, I wasn't feeling it; I was just a bit achy, but I assumed it was just usual post-exercise muscle stiffness.

But at 3.45am on 13 May, at 38 + 4 weeks pregnant, I was woken by what felt like a mild period cramp, and I soon realised that was happening every 10 minutes and they were contractions. Within the hour, the 30-second cramps were coming every 5 minutes. I suddenly needed to do two poos in quick succession, which can be a sign of early labour – this is because of the release of the prostaglandin hormone, which affects the smooth muscle in the womb and bowel, causing both to contract. But it's also because when the baby's head is low down and pushing through the birth canal, it presses the stretch receptors in the bowel, stimulating the sacral nerve and sending a message to the brain that you need to open your bowels.

At 5.30am I decided it was probably time to wake Rupert and let him know what was happening. At that point, the contractions weren't too bad and, as they lasted such a short time, they were manageable. I WhatsApped the midwives to let them know this was happening. They hadn't seen the message, but I wasn't worried, after all, the first stage of labour in first-time pregnancies can take hours, if not days. At 6am I did another poo, but then saw some vaginal blood. There was no mucus but I assumed it had just come out in the toilet with the poo and that this was my 'show', and off went another WhatsApp to the midwives.

By 7am the contractions were coming every 2 minutes and lasting 45 seconds; they were also intensifying, so I took paracetamol, started the TENS machine up and Rupert called the midwives. They didn't seem worried and said that it's not uncommon for first-time mums to have contractions that start and then stop for 24 hours, then come back tomorrow or last for days. Rupert passed the phone to me and they said that as I was able to talk through the contractions that I would be fine just to continue to monitor and let them know if it became more regular or intensified. This was a bit of a blow to me as it was pretty bloody intense at that point. They suggested we start getting the birthing pool ready but not to fill it as it was too soon. I was also advised to try to sleep, watch a movie or eat to keep my strength up for the upcoming intensities. There was no chance I could sleep through these contractions; the mere suggestion felt a little insulting! Instead, we put *Superbad* on and Rupert made me a bowl of cereal, but by 8am we were having to pause the movie every 2 minutes due to minute-long contractions. Rupert got to inflating the birth pool, and I filled a warm bath to help me.

At 8.45am I was sitting in the bath, thinking 'this is getting unbearable', when suddenly there was a pinkish release of water. Was this my waters breaking? Off went another WhatsApp 15 minutes later, a lot of blood was coming out and I got scared. I tried to use my rationale doctor's hat, but my maternal animal hat was on instead, worried that my darling baby was coming to harm. Rupert called the midwives and they said they could be with me by 9.50am.

By this point the pain was crazy and it felt like my vagina was ripping. At 9.15 I felt something coming out of my vagina and I freaked out that it was the head; I couldn't see over my massive bump, so I asked Rupert to take a look, but he said it was more white-coloured and 'looked like an ostrich egg'. I realised this was probably the amniotic sac, and possibly the waters hadn't broken after all, or it was just trickling (that big gush of water you tend to see in the movies rarely happens!). Knowing this was coming out, I knew the baby was coming too!

I had the sudden urge to push. Nothing could have stopped me. Not all the reading I had done about protecting my perineum and 'gentle blowing motions' could stop this primal urge. Four of the most excruciating pushes later and at 9.24am there was a baby's head and I was standing in the bath telling Rupert to catch it! He caught it like a rugby ball; I sat back down, he passed it to me and I told him to call the ambulance. I put our baby against my chest to keep it warm and begged that it would start to cry, it did, almost instantly! On the phone, 999 told him to give me lots of towels to wrap the baby with and keep us warm. I was sitting in a bath full of blood and didn't care because my baby was breathing. While Rupert was on the phone, it dawned on me that I didn't check its sex! A boy!! A beautiful boy. I told Rup, and he looked so worried and thrilled in equal measure.

For a glorious 15 minutes we were all alone, a brand-new family of three. Clueless but ecstatic. Then the ambulance arrived, they checked Harris, then me, then clamped the cord. In my birth plan I had wanted to check that the cord had stopped pulsating before they clamped it, but by this point my birth plan seemed a million lifetimes away. I could only assume that as it had been 20 minutes since his birth that it probably would have. I remember thinking that the paramedic seemed nervous clamping it, I think she hadn't done it many times, and her hands were shaking. I thought about all the times I had been a medical student or a very junior doctor and feigned confidence. But she did it, and she did it well, and Rupert, who is entirely scared of blood, needles and anything vaguely medical, cut the cord! I still laugh to this day about how Rupert once said to me whilst I was pregnant that he didn't really want to be 'down at the business end' during the labour and that what actually happened was he was the only one at the business end!

By about 10am, the midwives had arrived. I was still in the bath with Harris but the water had been drained. My bum and vagina were throbbing, having been sitting on hard porcelain for over 40 minutes. The paramedics wanted to take a few more readings of my blood pressure as it was low, but eventually they let me get up, and I went to the spare room carrying my darling Harris. I cannot remember at what point Harris started breastfeeding, whether it was in the bath whilst he was lying on my chest, or if it was when we got to the bedroom. But I recall him literally crawling his way to my nipple! He was a pro, there was nothing else I had to do. Well, nothing except go on to deliver the placenta.

I opted for an unaided delivery of my placenta, which means I did not receive the injection that aids the shrinkage of the womb to pull away at the placenta. Instead, we just waited whilst breastfeeding, allowed a natural release of oxytocin to contract the womb and push out the placenta. It took around an hour, and the midwives laid a gentle hand on my tummy and put a bit of traction on the cord by pulling it, and – boom – out of my vagina came a huge, bloody slug. It felt like such a welcomed pressure release when it came out, as though finally my body was mine again. Once that came out the paramedics could leave. The midwives then went sifting through the placenta that lay like an elephant's liver on my bedroom floor, looking to ensure it was all intact and there was nothing potentially still left inside me.

The joys continued when I then had to be checked for tears – two first-degrees to the bilateral labia and one second-degree in the posterior wall. I was borderline for needing stitches, but I opted against it, having decided that I'd done the rest of the labour without any intervention, so why start now? After the rest of the baby checks and ensuring I felt confident with breastfeeding, we were left alone with baby Harris.

Having had my first contraction at 3.45am, less than 9 hours later, the three of us lay in bed eating the snacks I had prepared to feed me through days of labour, watching the rest of *Superbad* and staring at our brand-new baby!

RUPERT'S STORY

I thought it would be funny to ask Rupert to write out his recollection of the day, assuming it would be a few lines long and would be a humorous anecdote about how different our perceptions are. But I was stunned when he sent me this gem of a piece, and it reminded me of how important this day is to your partner, too:

It was the height of lockdown one, and Sara and I elected to have a home birth. We desperately wanted to stay together during and after the labour. I'm not great under pressure, but I thought this was the best option; at the time, the Covid rules stated that partners could only be in the delivery room for about an hour after the birth, and neither of us were keen on that.

The night before was uneventful, Sara was pretty huge by this point, and it was that sticky May heat, so, to ensure we could both sleep without boiling up, we were in separate rooms.

From my recollection, Sara came down at about 6am and woke me saying, 'Something's happening', with a cheeky/nervous smirk on her face. Instant butterflies. At this point, our midwives had informed us that this being our first pregnancy, the labour would be a long one, 'At least an 18-hourer' (correct me if I'm wrong, Sara, it's been a long 3 years).

Sara sent them a quick WhatsApp bringing them up to speed, and they reassured us (I've just found the WhatsApp messages), *'Oh, it'll be hours, do feel free to get the pool blown up and the room set up to be all cosy, it sounds like it might be a little soon to fill the pool with water. Eat some meals and drink plenty, so you have some fuel on board! And maybe cuddle up and watch a film together to see if you can get a nap in.'* They were on the other side of London, so with that input, we settled in for a bit of *Superbad* and a snuggle in bed.

Fast-forward a couple of hours, the contractions started to speed up and Sara was experiencing what I perceived as discomfort. Note that when I say discomfort, I'm the type of guy that whines when he gets a splinter and flinches when Mummy tries to take it out with a pin. She'd been a trouper and hadn't had pain medication; the midwives were equipped with gas and air. We only had a couple of paracetamol in the house, and something called a TENS machine, which is like a mild taser for your stomach. Fingers crossed for the hypnobirthing training and the antenatal classes we'd done over Zoom.

I'd blown up the birthing pool on the kitchen floor, think paddling pool XL. I didn't want to fill it with warm water using the hot water tap and a hose for fear it would have cooled by the time we needed it; after all, we were in this for the long run.

Tea at the ready (decaf for Sara), I wandered back upstairs and started pacing; I'm a bit of a pacer. Unhelpful.

By about 8:30am, the contractions were getting more frequent, but Sara remained calm and collected; we messaged the midwives again, expressing a bit more urgency this time. Same kind of response: 'It's your first, this is all normal, and we predict that it'll be ages yet.' They suggested running an ordinary bath, so I got busy with that. By about 8:45am, Sara was nestled in the tub, with me perched next to it; the contractions started in earnest, and some blood started coming out into the bath. The water reminded me of rosé. Sara did a bit of squatting, this is not a massive bath, and I felt really sorry for her; she looked so uncomfortable; it was too late for the birthing pool – timelines had massively sped up. I started grabbing towels; I know it sounds corny, but I must have had about ten at the ready.

Sara was blowing hard and asked me to take a look and see what was happening, I'm not great with blood and gore IRL, and when I looked underneath, there was what I can only describe as an ostrich egg poking about two inches out; it was a shock. I mentioned this to Sara, and the cool head among us told me the baby was still in the birthing sac. I then got on the phone with the midwives; it was about 9am now – I expressed a modicum of urgency might be required, and they told me they'd be here in an hour.

I'd braced my arm over the bathtub and held onto the taps. Sara was using my arm as a chew toy, but it was the least I could do. I think the teeth marks disappeared after about a fortnight. And then Sara excelled, pushing for all she was worth, the odd scream here and there, an un-requested wake-up call for the neighbours; our dividing walls aren't that thick.

Sara was squatting in the bath for about another half an hour – excellent core strength, my wife! The 'egg' was almost out, and I prepared for the catch of my life; I played rugby at school but was by no means accomplished. I did not want the baby to hit its head on the bath, and I wasn't sure how slippery birthing sacs or newborns are (I forgot to Google that). Sara had fulfilled her role with aplomb; I only had to do this. Placing my hands underneath her and praying to Will Carling, I held out for what was to come, and then the baby plopped out; I'd caught it, and Sara fell back into the water, exhausted, and the next minute was a blur. I put the baby in Mum's arms and started piling on the towels. More towels, that'll make everything all right…

Then 999, I might have been babbling, can't precisely remember, maybe Sara recalls. I told them our address, that we'd delivered a baby at home and that the midwives wouldn't be here for about 45 minutes. Could they possibly send an ambulance?

999 operator: 'What sex is the baby?'
Me: 'Er, not sure.'
Sara: (peeking under the mountain of towels) 'It's a boy!'
Me: 'It's a boy!'

Then there was just relief and the most beautiful photo I'll ever take of Sara and baby Harris lying in the bath, surrounded by towels, with a smile on her face that will always melt my heart. Poor Sara was damaged down below and must have been in incredible pain, but she didn't show it. We were just both so happy. The ambulance arrived bang on time, and they let me cut the cord – squeamishness be damned.

Then back to bed and *Superbad*, Harris' first movie.

WHAT CAN BRING ON LABOUR?

Hurrah, you're finally 40 weeks pregnant, but where is your baby? Remember that term is technically up to 42 weeks, so you may just need to wait a bit longer. Wait longer? Easier said than done when you're not entirely convinced you can stretch anymore, and you have images of your baby trying to rip its way out of your stomach like in the movie *Alien*. So you turn to the internet in search of ways to bring on labour and you are faced with foods, activities and drinks, but which are evidence-based and which are just old wives' tales?

Walking – staying active in pregnancy has many benefits, and during the later weeks walking may help to bring on labour by keeping your body upright and helping the baby move downwards towards the cervix. Totally anecdotally, I put my early and quick labour down to doing pregnancy-friendly high-intensity interval training (HIIT) classes and yoga up until the day of my labour.

Eating dates – the suggestion of one very small study is that dates help stimulate the release of oxytocin, which helps to reduce the duration of labour and encourages birth closer to the due date[76]. However, larger, more robust studies are required to confirm this. But dates are so tasty, I feel it's worth a shot!

Drinking raspberry leaf tea – it is thought to 'tone' the womb, however, studies have not proven that it can induce labour. I did find a small study that found raspberry tea shortened the second stage of labour by 10 minutes and decreased the need for forceps[77].

Sex – it might be the last thing you fancy doing whilst you are in beached-whale mode, but in theory it may progress labour in two ways. Firstly, semen contains prostaglandins, which help to soften the cervix. Secondly, having sex releases the 'love' hormone oxytocin, which is needed for womb contractions. The prostaglandins and oxytocin will not trigger a labour, but they may help along a labour that has already started.

Spicy food – the idea is that the spicy food will stimulate your bowels and in turn your womb! There is no evidence for this, but you're welcome to try it if you fancy a nice little takeaway, though be aware of the potential for heartburn.

Acupuncture – acupuncture involves the insertion of fine needles into specific points of the body, and it has been stated as helping to soften and dilate the cervix with onset of labour contractions. NICE states that the available evidence does not support acupuncture for induction of labour[78]. The evidence does not reliably determine whether it will increase the chance of labour, but two trials have shown that it may promote a 'more favourable state of the cervix within 24 hours'[79].

Eating pineapple – both pineapple and papaya contain the enzyme bromelain, which is the chemical that can give your mouth that tingling sensation after you've eaten it, but bromelain has also been thought to soften the cervix and trigger contractions. However, the research is lacking, with only some rat studies suggesting contractions[80] (primarily when the pineapple was directly put on the womb rather than consumed) and not cervical softening, and none of them suggesting induction of labour[81]. So enjoy your pineapple for its wonderful tropical taste but don't expect bromelain or pineapple to actually have an inducing effect.

Nipple stimulation – this mimics the effects of a suckling baby and causes the release of oxytocin, which can trigger contractions. A meta-analysis found nipple stimulation resulted in a significant reduction in the number of women not in labour at 72 hours[82]. Most research studies performed this manually (with your fingers), but you can also stimulate your nipples using a pump or ask your partner to have a go at suckling (pre-warn them, they may get some colostrum!).

INDUCTION OF LABOUR

Labour does usually eventually start on its own, but in one in five pregnancies, labour is induced[83]. This is when the doctors or midwives artificially encourage the labour process to start.

The most common reasons for induction are:

- You have gone past 41 weeks of pregnancy – this is the most common reason for an induction.
- You or your baby have a medical problem – for example, diabetes, high blood pressure, intrahepatic cholestasis of pregnancy.

- There is a risk for your baby – for example, if you are over 37 weeks pregnant and your waters have broken with no signs of labour.

The first point can divide a room. As mentioned, term is actually 42 weeks, so offering everyone an induction at 41 weeks may feel a little premature. The national recommendation was brought down from 42 weeks to 41 weeks in 2021 based on research that compared induction times and showed higher infant mortality after 42 weeks if the woman had not been induced[84]. The rationale is that when pregnancies continue past 41 weeks there is an increased likelihood of having a C-section, baby needing admission to a neonatal Intensive Care Unit (ICU), and stillbirth or neonatal death. You read these things, and your natural instinct is probably to shout 'sign me up for an induction'! But it is important to consider a number of things when being offered one.

Firstly, understand what the relative and absolute risks are. Whilst it may very well be that the likelihood of these negative outcomes increase over time with a prolonged pregnancy, the absolute risk remains low. For example, if it is phrased that pregnancies after 43 weeks are over five times more likely to result in a stillbirth compared to at 37 weeks, you may feel an intense desire to be induced. But if you hear that the absolute risk is actually 10.8 in 10,000 versus 2.1 in 10,000[85], you may think, that's still an overall low risk, I'd like to wait a bit longer.

Secondly, recognise that when you hear that an induction lowers the chance of a stillbirth, it can depend on personal circumstances. This claim actually depends on the reason for induction. There are some very serious conditions whereby this intervention can save the life of both mother and baby, and if these are the reasons that you are being offered the induction, it would be wise to take heed. However, sometimes induction is being offered simply due to a theoretical risk factor, rather than basing it on your individual circumstances and clinical picture.

Thirdly, remember that stillbirth is not the only way to measure harm, and you need to discuss the potential harms that induction can cause. You may find that the minimal improvement in stillbirth rates in induction may not outweigh the side-effects and other risks[86]. For example, some studies have suggested higher neonatal mortality rates (from birth until 28 days postpartum), including Sudden Infant Death Syndrome (SIDS)[87].

Finally, understand what the impact of having an induction may have on your birth plans. Birth plans are not set in stone, and you need to be flexible for your and your baby's safety. However, if you were certain you wanted a water birth in the birthing centre, then having an induction will affect that. Studies have found that when labour is induced with pharmacological methods, 15 per cent went on to require further intervention in instrumental births (see assisted birth, page 110) and 22 per cent had emergency Caesareans[88]. Conversely, there will be some women who decide against the induction as they really hoped for a spontaneous birth, but still do not progress even with the added time and then require an emergency Caesarean. So, if you are keen to have a vaginal birth it is also worth taking this into consideration.

None of these facts are here to scare you, but simply to be informative. It is important to know all the pros and cons before deciding whether induction is right for you, and this may help you open up some talking points with your midwife or doctor *before* the time comes so that *if* the time comes, you can calmly and confidently make a decision.

If you have reached 41 weeks and your midwife has suggested booking in your induction, don't panic. You can book it and then change your mind. You can book it and go through with it. You can say no, and then change your mind and say yes. Or you can say no and ask to wait longer. You can also say no and ask for increased monitoring to ensure your baby's health through a cardiotocography (CTG), a continuous electronic record of the baby's heart rate obtained via an ultrasound transducer placed on your tummy or more ultrasound scans. You are the ruler of your body. Take advice, weigh the risks and benefits, and decide for yourself in your own time.

The questions I recommend you ask your healthcare provider to help you make the decision are as follows:

- Why is an induction being offered to me?
- When and where will this induction be carried out?
- What are the proposed induction methods?

- What are the arrangements for pain relief?
- What are the risks and benefits of induction in *my* specific circumstances?
- What are my options if the induction isn't successful?
- What are my alternative options if I don't want an induction?

HOW IS LABOUR INDUCED?

Let me begin by describing what happens naturally. The growing baby and the maturing placenta trigger the release of the hormone prostaglandin, which prepares the cervix (neck of the womb) for effacement and dilation. Effacement is the cervix's softening, thinning and shortening, while dilation is the opening. Then a rise in oestrogen levels and a decrease in progesterone make the womb more sensitive to oxytocin. The baby starts to migrate into the pelvis, and contractions kick off the effacement and dilation process. So labour begins when the baby, the mother, and her womb, placenta and hormones are ready.

Induction of labour works by trying to mimic these processes artificially. There are a few different stages to induction, but you may not need to have all of them. The first thing you may be offered is a 'sweep'; this is not technically part of the induction stages, but it is an intervention to get labour going, so I include it here. This is when the doctor or midwife places a finger inside the cervix and makes a circular sweeping motion with the aim of separating the amniotic membranes (the sac surrounding your baby) from the cervix, triggering the release of prostaglandins, which can increase your chance of entering labour within 48 hours. This involves no medications and is a fairly simple procedure that is carried out during an antenatal appointment. It can feel uncomfortable, and some people get light bleeding following the procedure, but this is not harmful to your baby. There are some cases in which a sweep is not offered that includes if your waters have already broken, if your baby's head is not down, if you have a low-lying placenta or if you've had significant bleeding during your pregnancy.

Another form of outpatient induction that one can be offered is the 'balloon'. This involves a catheter (soft silicone tube) being inserted into the cervix. The catheter has a balloon at the tip, which is then filled with sterile water once it is in place and can stay there for 24 hours. You can go home with this in place, and you return the following day for removal. It puts gentle pressure on the cervix, which causes the release of prostaglandin to help soften and open the cervix up. It may be an uncomfortable procedure, but it shouldn't be painful, and you can ask for gas and air if you need it.

The next stage for labour induction is to offer a gel, tablet or pessary that you insert into your vagina containing a synthetic version of the hormone prostaglandin, which helps prepare the cervix. This will happen on the maternity wards. Depending on whether you were given the immediate or slow-release version, you might expect to start contractions up to 6 hours or 24 hours later. You will be offered another dose if you have not started having contractions.

Following the softening of the cervix with the prostaglandins, the midwife may offer an artificial rupture of membranes, also known as breaking the waters. The midwife will make a small cut in the amniotic sac to release the waters.

If contractions have not started yet, you are then offered an intravenous drip containing the hormone oxytocin to help start contractions. This synthetic form of oxytocin can cause contractions that become stronger more quickly than naturally occurring contractions, so it is given at a very slow rate. To ensure that the contractions do not become too stressful for the baby and the womb, you are connected up to continuous electronic foetal monitoring. This anchoring with the monitoring and the IV line can make movement a bit more difficult and can feel frustrating, but, if it is all fitted securely, you can still ask to sit on a birthing ball, beanbag or chair if that is your preference.

Furthermore, induced labours can feel more painful than naturally induced labours. This can be because of the intensity of the contractions brought on by the synthetic oxytocin, but also because the synthetic oxytocin does not cross the blood–brain barrier, so this means that the brain does not get informed about the rise in oxytocin and therefore does not release the endorphins in response to the contractions. Endorphins act as our body's natural painkillers, so induced women may not benefit from them in helping to manage their contractions and may require further pain relief. The 2019 NHS survey of women's experiences of maternity care found that women whose labour was induced were more likely to have an epidural than women who had a spontaneous birth: 47 per cent of women whose labour was induced compared with 19 per cent of women who had a spontaneous birth[89].

If these induction methods do not result in labour and your baby's birthing, the options include a further attempt to induce labour, or a Caesarean section.

'Should I have an induction?' is a highly personal question, and it would likely depend on a number of factors, including your health and social circumstances, the hospital's policies, the risks to you and your baby, as well as how you manage uncertainties and previous experiences. If you feel that induction is the right thing for you and your baby, then say 'Yes' with the informed knowledge of what it entails. I didn't require an induction, so I don't know what I would have done had I crept towards the 42-week mark, but despite being a woman in science, my feelings are usually that nature trumps science. Nature is not perfect by any means, but what if we didn't have to spend those extra days over 41 weeks panicking about the prospect of induction and instead spend them delighting in the miracles of a maturing baby? In these last weeks, the baby grows, stores up body fat to help with temperature regulation, builds up their iron stores, improves their sucking and swallowing co-ordination and matures their lungs. We also continue to pass antibodies onto our babies that will help them fight infections. This slow and steady preparation for labour and the outside world is incredible, and if you feel that you need more time in that space and there is no clear medical indication that waiting will do more harm than good, you can make an informed decision to say 'no'.

THE STAGES OF LABOUR

Dividing labour into stages makes the process of giving birth to a baby all sound very orderly and civilised, but please remember that each body and each birth is different, and what happens in these stages can be experienced very differently from person to person. Some people may have a very short first and latent stage and move straight to the active and transition stage, and some may feel like they're in the latent stage forever!

FIRST STAGE OF LABOUR

This is usually the longest stage, when the cervix dilates up to 10cm (think the diameter of a melon – eek). This stage can be further divided into the latent, active and transition phases.

Latent phase

This is the first part of your labour, which can last several days and prepares your body for labour. During this phase the muscles in your womb contract, making the cervix shorter, thinner and softer. The cervix also moves into a more anterior (forward) position within the pelvis and starts dilating.

What symptoms might you experience in the latent phase? You may experience a number of symptoms during this phase. Contractions can be mild, period-like cramps to more severe contractions, they may last for hours and then stop, only to return again the following day, and they might be irregular. This start/stop pattern in the latent phase is common, especially in first-time mums. Every woman has a different pace and rhythm. You may also notice a 'show', which is a mucusy plug that can come away from your cervix as it becomes softer and shorter, and can sometimes contain streaks of blood. You may need to open your bowels several times. It may be during this phase that your waters break, though it can occur at any time during your labour. This is when the amniotic sac within which your baby develops breaks, releasing the amniotic fluid through your vagina. It is an odourless fluid, in a clear or pale straw colour. Movies will have you believe there is huge gush of water, and whilst that can be the case for some, for many it can also just feel like a popping sensation followed by a trickle, like you've peed yourself. The part of the amniotic sac that breaks has no pain receptors, so it will not hurt.

What should you do in the latent phase? This is the time when you should try to remain gently active, if possible, and eat to give you energy for the remaining labour. You can also do things that make you happy, to increase your oxytocin levels – perhaps put on a funny movie, invite close friends around, listen to a banging playlist or have a massage. If the contractions are causing you pain, you may find a warm bath helps, or you can consider taking a painkiller like paracetamol, which is safe in pregnancy, or put on your TENS machine. If your waters have broken, you may want to wear a pad, then you can observe the colour, smell and volume of fluid. You should also inform your midwife, who may want you to come in for an assessment.

Active phase

Once your cervix has dilated to 4cm (the diameter of a banana, for reference), we are in the active phase.

What symptoms might you experience in the active phase? Your labour tends to progress more quickly when you are in this phase. Your contractions will become more regular, stronger and closer together. A general rule of this phase is that you will experience regular and strong contractions that last around 60–90 seconds, every 3 to 4 minutes for at least an hour.

What should you do in the active phase? At this point you usually want to be seen and assessed by your midwife. If your cervix isn't 4cm yet, you will be sent back home and advised to wait for the contractions to become regular, stronger and closer together. If it is your first baby, this active phase of labour usually lasts around 8 hours and rarely exceeds 18 hours. If you have had a baby before, this is usually around 5 hours, rarely exceeding 12 hours. I must remind you that this is only an average; as you will have read from my birth story, my active phase only lasted an hour! If you are in active labour, then cue the birth plan! Your midwife will discuss pain relief with you here, monitor your baby's heartbeat, check your frequency of contractions, measure your blood pressure, pulse and temperature, check how often you need to pass urine and offer vaginal examinations to assess the progression of your labour.

Transition phase

At the end of the active phase of labour, between the first and second stages of labour, is the transition phase, which marks the end of the 'hanging out in the hospital' and the beginning of 'Oh my god, here we go.' By now your cervix will have dilated from 8 to 10cm.

What symptoms might you experience in the transition phase? It can feel like a very intense phase as there is a natural spike in adrenaline. It can make some women suddenly feel more emotional or out of control. The contractions are usually strong and you may start to feel the urge to push. Some women feel shaky, hot/cold or nauseous, and some even vomit.

What should you do in the transition phase? Some people go through this phase barely noticing it, whereas others feel entirely overwhelmed. If you are the latter, try to stay calm. During the adrenaline spike, some women feel like they want to give up, turn and run away. Others start to wail, moo and yell. Warn your partner about this phase beforehand and advise them to say supportive and kind things to you, even whilst you threaten them! It's all the adrenaline speaking, after all. Although it is a challenging phase, it is the shortest one, usually lasting 15 minutes to 1 hour.

SECOND STAGE OF LABOUR

This means your cervix is fully dilated at 10cm, and your baby is moving down through your vagina. Your body has changed from an opening-up phase to a bearing-down phase.

What happens in the second stage of labour? This second stage can be divided into passive and active. Passive simply means you do not yet have the urge to push along with the contractions yet, and active means you do. If you are a first-time mum, you are likely to give birth within 3 hours of the active second stage and 2 hours if you have had a baby before.

What symptoms might you experience in the second stage of labour? Your contractions will continue and may become stronger and longer, though they may also become more spaced out, allowing the mother a well-needed rest.

You usually feel the overwhelming urge to bear down and push during this stage. As the baby moves down the birth canal, the pressure is first felt on the rectum, so that you may feel more pressure in your bottom. If you are feeling panicked that you might open your bowels, well, you might, but it is entirely normal. The midwives and doctors expect it and will manage it swiftly and without issue. After all, how can you expect to push an entire baby out of you if you can't push out a poo? The head of the baby continues to descend and causes a stretching or burning sensation in the vagina and perineum as the skin stretches to its full capacity. This pain signals the mother to ease back on the pushing so that the skin can stretch gently around the crowning head. Your midwife will help guide you through this pushing process.

What should you do in the second stage of labour? Find a comfortable position to give birth in. Whilst it is commonly depicted in movies as a lying on your back process, in practice it tends to be more comfortable to labour in an upright or side-lying position. The gravity of upright positions helps your baby on its descent and the side-lying position allows more flexibility in your pelvis. In a meta-analysis, the researchers reviewed the results of 12 randomised controlled studies with a total of 4,314 labouring women, who were assigned to either an upright or a recumbent birth[90]. They found that the upright birthing positions led to a lower rate of instrumental delivery, a shorter (by 8 minutes) active pushing phase (16 minutes if squatting), and a lower risk of severe perineal trauma (though if squatting or using a birth seat this risk went up, but the rates of episiotomies went down). There was no difference in the blood loss between the groups and no difference in the total length of the second stage of labour. Ultimately, you need to feel comfortable and supported, and you have the right to be in whichever position you choose. If you have an epidural, you may prefer a lying-down position if it is a particularly 'heavy' dose, and if you are having foetal monitoring done it may be easier for the caregiver to attach this whilst lying down, but it should not be a deal breaker if you want to be upright. As described above, during this stage you will also have the urge to push with the contractions. Listen to your body, you will instinctively know when to push and when to rest, and your midwife will guide you through your breathing and pushing to allow your baby's head to come through slowly and gently to reduce the risk of tears.

THIRD STAGE OF LABOUR

You have your baby! Yay! So you're thinking, what 'third stage'!? Well, this is when you pass the placenta through your vagina. This can be done actively or passively.

Active management

A synthetic version of oxytocin is injected into your thigh, which stimulates further contractions. Whilst your contractions are occurring, your midwife will gently pull on the cord and deliver the placenta. It is important to deliver the placenta soon after administering the injection, to reduce the risk of a retained placenta. The pros of doing this are that the risk of postpartum haemorrhage and/or needing a blood transfusion is lower, and you are likely to deliver the placenta within 30 minutes. The cons of this are that there may be side-effects of nausea, vomiting, afterpains and a rise in blood pressure.

Physiological management

Whilst it is the national guideline that women have active management due to the lower risks of bleeding, physiological management is also a viable option. This is where no external action is taken to deliver the placenta. You will be advised to sit in an upright position. Your uterus will contract, and when the placenta drops into the vagina, you will feel a heaviness. Some women feel the urge to push, but others deliver it spontaneously. Often, breastfeeding and skin-to-skin contact helps to increase your oxytocin levels and may speed up the process, which can take up to an hour. If it takes longer than an hour or you're experiencing significant bleeding, you will be advised to have the injection.

Anything that inhibits the amount of natural oxytocin you produce can affect whether physiological management will work for you. This can occur in inductions, epidural use and specific pain relief. Oxytocin can also be inhibited in those who may have had a psychologically distressing labour or an excess of adrenaline release. Remember that you can always opt for physiological management and then change your mind and ask for the injection.

Cord clamping

As part of the third stage of labour, you will need to have the cord that attaches the baby's umbilicus to the placenta clamped and then cut. Even after your baby has been born, the cord continues to pulsate, transferring all the blood, oxygen and stem cells to your baby. It is recommended that the cord is not cut earlier than after 1 minute, to help transfer enough iron to keep baby topped up until they are 6 months old, and enough stem cells needed for their growth and immune system. It has also been shown to have some benefits for preterm babies, with fewer suffering from low blood pressure, requiring transfusions and a reduced risk of intraventricular haemorrhage (bleeding in the brain).

The time it takes for the cord to stop pulsating and transferring the blood to the baby can vary from 1 minute to 60 minutes. If you opt for active management of your placenta, the cord is usually clamped within 5 minutes to allow for the separation of the placenta from the womb. It tends to be done earlier to reduce any blood loss associated with the third stage. If you are having a physiological management of the placenta, the cord clamping can be delayed further until the placenta has been delivered or until it has stopped pulsating and the cord has become white.

See cord clamping, page 133, for more information about the benefits and risks of early or delayed cord clamping.

CAESAREAN SECTION

Whilst the majority of women in the UK give birth vaginally, one in four will have a Caesarean section (C-section or CS)[91], this may be an elective choice – which means the decision to have the CS was made ahead of labour starting; or it might be an emergency – which is decided upon once labour has begun.

The most common reasons for an elective CS are multiple pregnancies (twins, etc.), the baby presenting in breech position, placenta praevia, pre-eclampsia and previous CS(s). In the UK your midwife or doctor will not usually recommend a CS unless there is a medical indication; however, provided you have carefully weighed up the risks and benefits, you are allowed to request a CS.

There are many non-medical reasons why a woman might want to have a CS, including a previously difficult or traumatic vaginal birth, anxiety about the complications or pain associated with a vaginal birth and a better sense of control. Whatever your reasons, it is best to discuss them early with your midwife to ensure you have all the factual information and support available. In the UK, vaginal delivery and CS are considered relatively safe, but, as with any intervention, there are potential risks. The risks to you include an infection of the wound or the womb, bleeding, blood clots (DVT) and damage to the bladder. A CS may also affect future pregnancies, particularly if you decide on a vaginal birth the next time, as the scar in your womb could open up (uterine rupture), or the placenta might abnormally attach, not allowing it to come away as it should (placenta accreta). Still, most women are able to go on to have normal deliveries.

The risks to your baby include accidental cuts to the skin and breathing difficulties. However, the latter is more prevalent in those born before 39 weeks and usually resolves within a few days. There also seems to be a minimal increased chance of babies born by CS dying within the first 28 days, with one in 2,000 babies born by CS, compared to one in 3,300 after a vaginal birth[92], though this may be confounded by the reason behind why the CS was chosen in the first place. The most common causes for an emergency CS are foetal distress, your labour not progressing, or excessive bleeding.

WHAT HAPPENS DURING A CS?

An elective CS will usually be planned at around 39 weeks to reduce the risk that the baby will need to go to a neonatal unit. A CS takes place in an operating theatre, so it may feel a little cold and sterile in there, with lots of bright lights, but you can certainly make it feel more relaxed by playing music. You are usually also allowed to bring someone with you, who will need to wear scrubs and sit by your side (at the head end!). Caesarean sections are usually carried out under spinal or epidural anaesthetic, which means you will be awake, but you will not feel any pain in the lower part of your body, though you may feel some pulling and tugging. You will also have an IV line and catheter inserted. A screen will be placed across your body so that you can't see what is happening, but your doctor and the nurses will keep you in the loop throughout, if you would like to know. A cut measuring around 10 to 20cm will be made horizontally across your lower stomach (they will shave the area just before), and your muscles will be pulled aside, then another cut is made into your womb, through which they will deliver your baby. The cord will be clamped and cut, and, after the standard checks of the baby, it will be passed to you for skin-to-skin contact. Oxytocin is then given via the IV drip to help the placenta contract and separate from the wall of the womb, reducing blood loss, and the placenta and membranes are delivered through the incision. You will then be stitched back up. The stitches used to close the womb will be dissolvable. The outer skin wound will be closed using non-dissolvable stitches or staples that your midwife must remove in 5 to 7 days. The whole procedure usually takes around 40–50 minutes. You are then transferred to the recovery room, where you will be monitored, provided you are stable and well, before being transferred to the post-natal ward.

TROUBLESHOOTING – WHAT CAN GO 'WRONG' IN LABOUR?

Wrong is not the right word here; this is more of a section on the possible different outcomes. But 'wrong' is how it can feel to a labouring mother who has an idea of how they want their birth to look, then suddenly find it is deviating far away from that plan. As you will have read from my birth story, it wasn't exactly as I planned; I had zero intentions of birthing my baby without a midwife. It was a little terrifying, but ultimately left me with the most extraordinary and incredible experience, though not one I plan on replicating anytime soon! I am not suggesting that you prepare yourself for a solo birthing, but still, I firmly believe that forewarned is forearmed, so if we can educate ourselves on all the possible variables beforehand, we may feel less overwhelmed and stressed if they become your birthing reality.

WATERS HAVE BROKEN EARLY

Most waters break during labour, but sometimes waters break early, which is known as premature rupture of membranes (PROM). If PROM occurs before 37 weeks of pregnancy, it is called preterm premature rupture of membranes (PPROM). The concern with PROM is an increased risk of infection to your baby, with the risk of a severe neonatal infection being 1 per cent (versus 0.5 per cent in women with intact membranes)[93].

If you are 37 weeks or more pregnant and your waters have broken, put a sanitary pad on so the midwives can observe the colour of the fluid coming out, and contact the midwives. They are likely to advise you to attend the hospital for an assessment. Labour usually starts within 24 hours of the waters breaking, so providing all is well with you and the baby, you may be advised to return home and wait for labour to commence.

Research suggests there is no greater risk to you or your baby if you go home versus staying in the hospital.[94] At home, you will be advised to check your temperature every 4 hours, and if you start to feel unwell, hot, feverish, or your temperature goes above 37.5 degrees, you will be advised to contact your midwife. You will also be advised to continue wearing a sanitary pad and to change it regularly, and use it to observe the waters. They may be a little bloodstained to start, but if you continue to lose blood or the waters become smelly, cloudy, green or brown, you need to inform your midwife immediately. If after 24 hours you have not gone into labour, you are likely to be offered an induction, and the health of you and your baby will be checked regularly. If your membranes were ruptured for more than 18 hours before your baby is born, it is usually recommended that you stay in the hospital for a further 12 hours afterwards to ensure no signs of infection in your newborn baby.

If you are under 37 weeks pregnant, the aim is to try to get you as close to 37 weeks as possible before giving birth. You should, as above, wear a sanitary pad and contact your midwives straight away for assessment. They will offer you antibiotics to reduce the risk of infection and will monitor for any signs of infection. Providing you and your baby are well, they may try to allow the pregnancy to continue. However, if you or your baby do develop signs of an infection or any other complication, you may need to give birth immediately.

ASSISTED DELIVERY

This simply means that the medical team needs to use specially designed instruments to help you deliver your baby. It might feel disappointing that you need intervention, but it is common, with around a third of first-time mums requiring an assisted delivery (it becomes less common with consequent pregnancies).

The most frequent reasons for being offered an assisted delivery are that there are concerns about your baby's wellbeing (they may be in distress or there are worries about its heart rate); the baby's position is awkward, not allowing for an easy transition through the birth canal; the labour isn't progressing as expected, and you have been pushing for a long time; or that you are unable to or have been advised against pushing during birth.

One of the instruments used is called a ventouse, also known as a vacuum cup. The small cup is placed on your baby's head, creating a vacuum so that when the healthcare provider pulls it whilst you push, it offers traction to help guide the baby out. Forceps are the alternative method, and are long, curved metal tongs that fit around the baby's head, which help the medical team pull on the baby during your contractions to help ease it out. Which you are offered can depend on the position of your baby, your specific circumstances and the gestational age of your baby. If you are less than 36 weeks pregnant, you tend to be offered the forceps over the ventouse, as the baby's head is still too soft at that age. If one method is tried and is not successful, it may be that you are offered the other method, or you may be offered an emergency Caesarean section. Assisted deliveries can usually continue in the room where you first went into labour, providing you are on a labour ward. If you are in a birthing centre, you will be transferred to a labour ward. Still, if it is thought that it may not be successful or there are any concerns about you or your baby's wellbeing, an assisted delivery may be carried out in the operating theatre so that if it is not successful you are in the right place for an emergency Caesarean section.

It has been found that assisted delivery is more successful in those with a BMI less than 30, a height greater than 161cm, an estimated baby weight of less than 4kg, a baby's position not in the occiput-posterior (the baby is head down with its back against your back, known as 'back to back'), and a baby whose head is low down in the birth canal.

During an assisted delivery, you will usually have a catheter inserted to empty your bladder. This small tube is passed through your urethra and into the bladder. You will then be offered pain relief if you have not had an epidural. You will likely require an episiotomy (see episiotomy, page 112) to allow for a larger opening to birth your baby.

The risks associated with an assisted delivery include a heavier bleed after birth, a greater risk of blood clots to your legs or pelvis, and an increased risk of a third- or fourth-degree tear (see perineal tear, page 112). Third- and fourth-degree tears affect 3 per cent of women who have vaginal births[95], but following a ventouse birth, this goes up to 4 per cent, and following a forceps birth, this can go up to between 8 and 12 per cent[96]. This degree of tear can result in increased anal incontinence. Urinary incontinence may also be more common after an assisted delivery. You will usually be offered antibiotics through an IV line to negate the risk of infection to you after an assisted delivery.

Regarding the risks to your baby, their head may be marked with superficial cuts or grazes, affecting 10 per cent of babies born with assisted delivery[97]. The ventouse cup usually leaves a swelling on the head, which disappears within 48 hours[98], and, in 1–12 per cent of babies, the forceps can leave a bruise (cephalohematoma), which will also disappear in time. Cephalohematomas can slightly increase the risk of jaundice in the first few days, which is where you get a build-up of a chemical called bilirubin that can cause yellowing to the skin and the eyes. Newborn jaundice is usually harmless and doesn't often need treatment. A paediatrician (children's doctor) is usually called to be at assisted deliveries to check on the child's wellbeing. Providing all is well, the baby can still be handed straight to you for skin-to-skin contact.

If you decide you do not want an assisted delivery, you can either continue to try to give birth without assistance, or you can opt for an emergency Caesarean section.

PERINEAL TEAR

On birthing your child, your vagina and perineum must significantly stretch to allow the baby's head to pass through and, on doing so, you may experience a perineal tear. Around 90 per cent of first-time mums will experience some sort of tear, and while for most women this may just be a small cut or graze that will heal on its own, for around a third of women in the UK, it might require stitches[99]. Perineal tears are graded by degree. A first-degree tear is just a small tear affecting only the skin, and it usually heals quickly without the need for any treatment. A second-degree tear affects the muscle as well as the skin, and usually requires stitches, and third- or fourth-degree tears are even deeper and can extend as far down to the anal sphincter (the muscle that controls the anus) and usually need to be repaired with surgery. Perineal tears tend to be a feared outcome, but they are common and, although they sound nasty, the vast majority heal well. Remember to read the section on perineal massage on page 75 to reduce your risk of perineal tears.

EPISIOTOMY

An episiotomy is when a midwife or doctor cuts the perineum (the area between the vagina and the anus) to allow for more space for the baby's head to come out. In the UK, episiotomies are not routinely practised and are only offered if a medical need exists. This includes if assistance in the form of forceps or ventouse is required to birth your baby, if your baby is in distress and they need to try to birth it with more ease, your baby is lying breech (that is, not head first), you are exhausted from pushing, or you have a medical condition that means you need to birth your baby quickly. The idea is that not only is it easier to birth your baby with the episiotomy, but the controlled episiotomy may prevent a more severe perineal tear.

If you need an episiotomy, you will be offered pain relief if you have not had an epidural, and a local anaesthetic can be applied. The cut made is a diagonal one downwards and to one side, and after the birth, it is stitched up again. After an episiotomy, it may be sore for a few weeks. It is important to keep the area clean, washing it regularly with water and changing pads regularly. It's also important to ensure your bowels are opening regularly by drinking plenty of water and eating a healthy diet with fibre, fruit and vegetables to avoid constipation. The stitches used are usually dissolvable, so you will not have to have these taken out.

'FAILURE' TO PROGRESS

I hate this terminology. Failure implies fault, of which, I want you to know, there is none. It means that the progression of your labour has slowed down, and it can occur at any stage of labour. Slow progression of labour may be considered if the cervix has dilated less than 2cm in 4 hours, if the progress of labour overall is slowing down, if the head of the baby is not descending and rotating, or if there are changes in the strength, duration and frequency of contractions.

You may be encouraged to change to an upright position, and your midwife will ensure good hydration and bladder emptying. You may be offered to have your waters broken if they haven't already, then be transferred to the labour ward if you are not already there, for care under the obstetrics team, where they will consider an oxytocin drip to stimulate contractions. If there are any concerns about the mother's or baby's health, the doctors may consider an assisted delivery or Caesarean section.

BABY'S POSITION

Most babies are born head first, as it is easier and safer in this position for your baby to pass through the birth canal. In one in 10 pregnancies, whilst the baby's head is down, it is in a posterior position, which means that the baby's head is facing your front instead of your back (so you are back to back). Most babies will turn at some point during the labour, but, where they don't, it can mean longer labour with back pain, and you may need an assisted delivery to help ease the baby round and out.

Breech position is when the baby presents their bottom or feet first, rather than the head. Around one in five babies are breech at 30 weeks pregnant, but most turn, so only three in 100 are still breech by the end of pregnancy[100]. The turning may happen on its own, but, once you reach 37 weeks, it is less likely they will turn on their own accord.

You may need to have an External Cephalic Version (ECV) to adjust the baby's position, where the doctor gently tries to coax the baby around by applying pressure on parts of your tummy. It can feel uncomfortable and sometimes painful, but the procedure should only last a few minutes. It may not be successful on the first attempt and, if so, you will likely be advised to return for further attempts. It has around a 40–60 per cent success rate and a low complication rate[101]. The most common complication is a transient change in the baby's heart rate, which is why your baby's heart rate is monitored throughout the procedure. In one in 200 babies, the ECV results in bleeding behind the placenta or damage to the womb, and they will need to be delivered by emergency Caesarean section immediately after. To assess for these complications, you will be monitored for symptoms including vaginal bleeding and abdominal pain and your baby will be monitored for fluctuations in their heart rate during the procedure. Uncommonly, five in 100 babies will manage to turn back around into a breech position after the ECV.

This is more 'out there' but there is also evidence that a moxibustion treatment may help your baby turn[102]. It is a traditional Chinese medicine that involves burning a herb called mugwort close to the acupuncture point BL67, located at the tip of your fifth toe. It can be used on pregnant women between 33 and 35 weeks and is commonly administered for 15–20 minutes a day for ten days, though there is no formal documented treatment regime. There are no known risks or side-effects to the mother or baby in using moxibustion.

Several factors can increase your risk of having a breech baby, including if this is your first baby, if you have a low-lying placenta, if you have too much amniotic fluid around your baby, or if you are having multiple births. You may read articles suggesting that moving yourself in certain positions may help your baby turn around, but no evidence supports this[103].

MECONIUM

Meconium is a newborn's first bowel movement, and it is sticky, thick and dark green. Babies usually pass it anytime in the first few hours to first few days following birth, however, some pass it in the amniotic fluid whilst they are still in the womb. Meconium in the amniotic fluid is more common if you are overdue.

If your midwife observes meconium in your amniotic fluid it can be a sign of foetal distress and can put your baby at risk of postnatal complications. As such, you may be transferred to the labour ward, if you are not already there, to monitor your baby's heart rate and contractions more closely. It causes no problems for most babies, but the main concern is that the baby might inhale some of the meconium and develop meconium aspiration syndrome, which causes respiratory distress.

If thick or lumpy meconium has been noted during labour, your baby will be assessed for signs of respiratory distress after birth. If there are any signs, your baby's airways may be cleared using suction. If your baby is entirely well, they will still need to be observed every 2 hours for 12 hours after the birth. If only a light meconium has been seen, your baby will likely only be checked 1 and 2 hours after birth[104]. If there are any concerns about your baby's condition, they will be reviewed by a paediatrician.

PRECIPITOUS LABOUR

This is also known as rapid labour – birthing your baby within 3 hours of your contractions starting. I know it might sound like a blessing to have a quick labour, but, when it happens that quickly, it can feel like you are going from zero to 100 without the intermediate time to get used to what is happening and to feel in control of the situation. As well as feeling overwhelming, a precipitous labour can also increase your risk of heavy postnatal bleeding, perineal tears and a retained placenta. You are at an increased risk of precipitous labour if you have had one before; if you have had one or more babies; high blood pressure; a baby with low birth weight and postpartum haemorrhage.

POSTPARTUM HAEMORRHAGE

Whilst it is normal to bleed after birth, heavy bleeding is known as postpartum haemorrhage (PPH) and requires urgent management. PPH can be further divided into primary and secondary. Primary PPH is when you lose 500ml or more of blood in the first 24 hours after birth. Secondary PPH is when you start having heavy bleeding between 24 hours and 12 weeks after birth.

If you have primary PPH and aren't already in a hospital, you will be transferred to a hospital. The midwife or doctor will try to encourage the womb to contract by massaging your womb through your abdomen or vagina, and they will also give you an injection of oxytocin into your thigh (if you already had one at birth, you will be given a second one). Placing a catheter tube in your bladder may also help the womb to contract. You will also have an IV line put in your arm to give you fluids, and you may be given an oxygen mask to wear. If your placenta hasn't already been delivered, the team will gently put traction on the cord to try to guide it out. If it has been delivered, they will check to ensure there aren't any missing pieces that could still be inside your womb that need to be removed. If bleeding continues, you may need a blood transfusion and further medication to get your blood to clot. If bleeding is still not under control, you may be transferred to the theatre for surgical input.

Several factors can put you at increased risk of a primary PPH, including placenta praevia, placental abruption, multiple births, pre-eclampsia/high blood pressure, previous PPH, BMI of over 35, anaemia, fibroids, clotting conditions, blood thinning medication, Caesarean section, induction of labour, retained placenta, perineal tear/episiotomy, assisted delivery, long labour (over 12 hours), large baby (heavier than 4kg), having your first baby over 40, fever during labour and needing general anaesthetic during labour.

Secondary PPH is usually caused by an infection in the womb or retained placenta in the womb. It will usually present with a bleed that becomes heavier or smellier, or you may start to feel unwell. It is usually treated with antibiotics, but if the bleeding persists, you may need IV antibiotics or have an operation to remove any retained placenta.

RETAINED PLACENTA

Sometimes, the placenta, or just part of it, remains in the womb after birth, which can cause the complication of postpartum haemorrhage. It is diagnosed if you haven't delivered the placenta within one hour of birth if you opted for physiological management or within 30 minutes if you opted for active management.

This can happen if the womb does not contract properly after birth, if the umbilical cord snaps, if the placenta has embedded particularly deeply into the womb, or if it has detached but is stuck behind a closing cervix. It is more common in women over 30 who have endured long labour, premature birth and stillbirth.

If you are not already in the labour ward, you will be transferred there, where you may be offered oxytocin to help your womb contract. You will also be encouraged to breastfeed, which can help your womb contract. A doctor may try to remove the placenta manually, but you may require surgery if these methods do not work.

PLACENTAL ABRUPTION

Placental abruption is when some or all of the placenta separates from the womb's wall before birth. The significance of this on your baby depends on the degree of separation and at what stage of the pregnancy it occurs. It can increase your risk of a premature birth, growth restriction and stillbirth. The symptoms of placental abruption include vaginal bleeding, abdominal pain, contractions and lower back pain, and if you experience these you should contact your midwife, maternity unit or GP immediately. If you are unable to get through to them, call 111 or 999 if the bleeding or pain is severe. If you are over 34 weeks pregnant when this occurs, you will be advised to give birth immediately, and if you or your baby are unwell, you may be advised to have a Caesarean section. If you are under 34 weeks and your baby is well, you will be monitored closely and advised to give birth by 37 or 38 weeks[105]. If you or your baby are unwell, you may have to have an immediate C-section.

ABNORMAL HEART RATE OF THE BABY

Your baby's heart rate can be monitored continuously using electronic foetal monitoring (EFM), or at intervals using intermittent auscultation. EFM works by placing two pads (transducers) on your stomach, which are held in place with two elastic belts. The transducers electronically send the information to the machine to produce a paper printout of the baby's heartbeat. Intermittent auscultation uses a device called a Pinard stethoscope, which is placed on your abdomen, and the midwife or doctor rests their ear on the other side, and will listen for at least a minute every 15 minutes once your labour is established. They may also use a small handheld ultrasound device. Providing you have an uncomplicated pregnancy and labour, there is no evidence to suggest that continuous monitoring is any more beneficial[106]; however, if there are any concerns, this may be switched to EFM. NICE recommends EFM if the baby is smaller than expected if you have high blood pressure, multiple births, a previous C-section, induced labour, are overdue or premature[107].

The normal heart rate of a foetus is between 110 and 160 beats per minute, and a variation can be caused by the womb contracting, limiting the blood flow to the placenta and, therefore, to your baby. Most babies can cope with these variations, but if the baby is not coping, it may be reflected in changes in the heartbeat. If this is the case, it may be that your baby will need to be delivered immediately via Caesarean section, or you may be offered foetal blood sampling first. It involves taking one or two drops of blood from your baby's scalp, which is then tested for oxygen levels and acidity, which will give a more accurate idea of how your baby is coping.

PERINATAL ASPHYXIA

This is when there is a lack of oxygen supply to your baby before birth. The cause is not always known, but the lack of oxygen can lead to brain injury. Possible causes include placental issues like abruption or placenta previa, umbilical cord compression or prolapse, conditions like pre-eclampsia and diabetes, and complications during labour and delivery. The extent of injury can range, with some babies experiencing no obvious long-term effect, and others suffering with severe disability.

Treatment involves immediate resuscitation to restore the oxygen supply and cooling therapy to limit the extent of brain injury.

Cooling therapy involves cooling the baby from the normal body temperature of 37°C down to 33.5°C for about 3 days. This is done using a special cooling wrap. After 72 hours of cooling, the baby's temperature is slowly returned to normal.

SHOULDER DYSTOCIA

This is when, during labour, one of your baby's shoulders becomes stuck behind your pubic bone, requiring extra help to release the shoulder and deliver the baby safely. It is considered an emergency, so if this occurs it is likely your midwife will call for assistance. You will be advised to stop pushing whilst you are placed into a different position (on your back with your legs pushed outwards and towards your chest), and your tummy will be pressed on. You may also have an episiotomy. If these don't help, you will be asked to go on all fours and the doctor or midwife will try to release the shoulder by placing their hand in your vagina.

It is difficult to predict when shoulder dystocia might occur but it can be more likely if you have had a baby with shoulder dystocia before, if you have diabetes, a BMI of more than 30, your labour is induced, you have a long labour, or you have an assisted birth.

One in 10 babies with shoulder dystocia will have a brachial plexus injury, where the nerves in the neck become stretched[108] and may cause a loss of movement to the arm, but this is usually temporary, lasting hours to days.

PAIN RELIEF

Oh God, how much will this hurt? I know that fear. It's every first-time mum's fear. However, it is not conducive to an easy birth. Our fight-and-flight response goes off when we are scared, which causes a surge in adrenaline and, conversely, inhibits the production of oxytocin, which we need for the progression of labour. Staying relaxed, safe and calm during labour will help ease the progression and, in turn, help you manage the pain better. For me, hypnobirthing helped me overcome that fear. I plastered my walls with positive affirmations about how my body was made to give birth, that I could cope with it, and that it would be a beautiful process that I had been gearing up to. It also helped that I was having a home birth in an environment I felt safe in and in company that I trusted. I asked for gas and air (Entonox), but, given the speedy circumstances of my birth and lack of midwives, I went through labour with paracetamol, bath and a TENS machine. I also utilised my husband's fleshy arm to bite on when the contractions were overwhelming! Knowing your pain relief options beforehand may take you halfway to feeling more in control, safe and confident in your coping abilities.

RELAXATION

There are many different relaxation methods, including breathing techniques, aromatherapy massage and meditation. While they may not remove your pain, they can aid as distractions and are easy to do anywhere. They tend to work better if they are started in the earlier stages of labour, to help you relax into active labour.

Massage – you do not need to hire a masseuse, but it can be helpful for your partner to learn basic massage techniques, which are usually taught in antenatal classes.

Breathing techniques – the theory behind these is based on the redirection of concentration so that during a contraction your thought processes are redirected from the pain to breathing instead. Mothers are usually taught deep abdominal breathing methods to help them to relax and act as a distraction. Often when we are anxious or upset, we breathe shallowly from the upper part of our chest, but, instead, taking slow, deep breaths from the abdomen is more beneficial. One way to know if you are achieving this is to place your hands along the bottom of your ribcage so that the fingertips of each hand are just touching, and as you breathe in, the fingertips should move apart slightly. Take deep, intentional and slow breaths, counting for 4 seconds as you breathe in and releasing the breath slowly for 4 seconds.

Sound therapy – this technique involves using soothing music or calming sounds to help create a peaceful environment during childbirth.

Aromatherapy – these essential oils can be used in massage, through a diffuser, in the bath (not in the birthing pool) or applied on a tissue or material to breathe in or on warm compresses. Some midwives are specifically trained in aromatherapy and can offer different blends if you do not have any medical conditions preventing its use. Several essential oils are traditionally used in labour, and the purported benefits of each are as follows. However, one must be mindful that there are not enough studies to confirm these alleged benefits in labour robustly:

- Clary sage is a natural painkiller that helps with regular contractions. (Not to be used in women with threatened premature labour, previous uterine surgery, or if labour is already well established.)

- Frankincense to help with anxiety.
- Jasmine and rose to help with anxiety and depression. (Not to be used in women with threatened premature labour or previous uterine surgery – avoid until term.)
- Lavender for anxiety, calming and relaxing.
- Lemon and mandarin for energy and mood boost.
- Peppermint for nausea and vomiting.
- Chamomile to help with anxiety (to be avoided until the third trimester).
- Grapefruit for anxiety.

The list is not limited to the above.

A meta-analysis pulling together the results of 17 studies showed that aromatherapy reduced labour pain in the transition phase and the duration of the active and third phases of labour, and was generally safe for mothers[109]. However, the analysis suggested that further trials, larger sample sizes and better-designed studies should be conducted before strongly recommending aromatherapy.

My thought pattern was that a bit of lavender in a diffuser was unlikely to cause me or the baby any harm, and may chill me out, so I bought one. It never made it out on labour day and sits sadly in a storage cupboard, but you never know when I will need it again for its anxiety-busting properties. Currently, NICE[110] states that aromatherapy should not be offered or advised for use as pain relief during the latent stage of labour, as there is limited evidence to support this at present, but if the woman wishes to use this technique, her wishes should be respected[111].

Water birth – the relaxing effect of warm water can boost your endorphin release, which is our body's natural painkiller. The buoyancy of the water also supports 75 per cent of the body's weight, which can aid comfort and allow for better mobility[112]. It has been found that women who have water births are less likely to go on to need epidurals and spinals and that the first stage of labour was reduced by an average of 32 minutes[113]. Whilst in the water, you can have Entonox, but you will not be able to have an epidural. Some of the injections can be given, but as they can make you drowsy, you will be advised to come out of the water and only return once the side-effects of the drug have worn off.

Movement/position – every time a contraction came on, I naturally, without thought, just shifted onto my knees and leaned forward with a rocking motion. This position takes the pressure off your back and allows the baby's head to continue to bear down on the cervix, promoting oxytocin release to dilate the cervix further. Birthing balls, bean bags and cushions can also help support a position that is comfortable for you.

TENS – a transcutaneous electrical nerve stimulation (TENS) machine is a small, battery-powered device that sends electrical currents through your body via sticky pads on your back and stimulates your nerves. It works by assisting your body to release endorphins and by disrupting the pain signals to the brain. The NICE guidelines suggest that it is likely only effective in early labour[114]. What I like about the TENS is that it gives you a sense of control over your pain relief, as you can press the 'boost' button every time you experience a contraction. It feels like a buzzing vibration on your back, which isn't painful or uncomfortable, but I didn't find it particularly pleasant either. I hadn't tested it out before labour and I think, in retrospect, I should have, so that I was expecting how it would feel.

MEDICATION

Entonox – also known as gas and air, is a mixture of nitrous oxide and oxygen. It is used in several procedures for short-term pain relief and anxiety. It is self-administered using a mouthpiece that gives you total control over when you need the relief and takes about 15–20 seconds to work, so you breathe in just as the contraction starts. It can make you feel tired, nauseous and lightheaded initially, but most women get used to the effect, and it will stop shortly after you stop using it. There are no known side-effects of Entonox to the baby.

Pethidine or diamorphine – these are injections usually given to you in your arm or leg that can take about 30 minutes to kick in and the effects of which will last a couple of hours. It can make you feel sleepy and slow down your breathing. If given too close to the delivery time, it can make your baby slower to breathe, and the drowsiness may also make them slower to feed at first. It is therefore not advised if you are nearing the second stage of labour.

Remifentanil – a small dose of Remifentanil can be given to you from a pump into an intravenous line in your hand. This is a patient-controlled pain relief, so you press a button to give yourself a dose every time you feel a contraction starting, and it usually kicks in within minutes. It can make you feel sleepy, sick and sometimes more breathless, so you will need to have a saturation probe on your finger to check your oxygen levels, and you may be given additional oxygen to breathe. This, too, may make your baby more slow to breathe initially, but its effects do not last long.

Epidural – a local anaesthetic (and often an opioid painkiller) is passed through a small tube that is inserted into your back. It numbs the pain signals carried from your birth canal to your brain, so it should offer complete pain relief. It can only be done and administered by an anaesthetist, who will ask you to lie curled on your side; they will clean the area with antiseptic and numb the skin with a local anaesthetic, then insert a needle into your back. A thin tube will be passed through the needle until it reaches the nerves in your back, and through this tube the medicine is administered. The needle is then removed. It can take up to 15 minutes for the pain relief to work. Occasionally the epidural needs to be adjusted or replaced. As you may no longer be able to feel the contractions, you can rely on your midwife to tell you when to push. This can prolong the second stage of labour and may increase the need for an assisted delivery. Low blood pressure and difficulty passing urine can be common side-effects, so you will also be given IV fluids to maintain your blood pressure, and you may also have a catheter inserted into your bladder. One in 100 women experience a headache[115], one in 1,000 women experience temporary nerve damage, often in the form of tingling or pins and needles in the legs, and one in 13,000 experience permanent nerve damage[116].

LABOUR: A TIRED MAMMA'S SUMMARY

STAGES OF LABOUR

- The first stage of labour, the longest, is divided into two phases: the latent phase and the active phase. During the latent phase, the cervix prepares for labour by becoming shorter, thinner and softer. Contractions begin, ranging from mild cramps to more intense contractions, and the cervix starts to dilate. In the active phase of the first stage, contractions become more regular, stronger and closer together. This is when a woman is usually seen by a midwife or healthcare provider for assessment.
- The transition phase marks the end of the active phase and the beginning of the second stage of labour. During this intense phase, the cervix fully dilates to 10cm, contractions are strong and the urge to push may arise.
- During the second stage of labour contractions continue, and the mother feels the urge to push. The head of the baby descends through the birth canal, causing pressure and stretching sensations. Different birthing positions are discussed, with upright positions generally showing advantages in terms of reduced intervention and perineal trauma risks.
- The third stage of labour focuses on delivering the placenta. This can be done actively with the help of synthetic oxytocin, or passively without external intervention. Delayed cord clamping is recommended, allowing the baby to receive vital blood and stem cells.

CAESAREAN SECTIONS

- Procedure where the baby is delivered through an incision made in the mother's abdomen and uterus. This might be an elective or emergency procedure.

COMPLICATIONS OF LABOUR

Premature rupture of membranes (PROM) – when the waters break early. Risks include the possibility of infection, monitoring and induction if necessary.

Assisted delivery – medical intervention is needed to aid in childbirth, such as forceps or ventouse delivery.

Perineal tear – the common occurrence of tears that occur in the perineum (area between vaginal opening and anus) during childbirth. These tears can range from minor to more severe, depending on the extent of the tissue damage. Most heal well, but some require intervention.

Episiotomy – a deliberate incision made in the perineum to create a controlled, planned opening to facilitate a smoother delivery. They are no longer routine and only offered if there is a medical indication.

Failure to progress – when labour progress slows down and potential interventions may be employed to stimulate labour.

Baby's position – abnormal foetal positions (not head down and facing your back), including breech presentation, can affect the ease of childbirth. External Cephalic Version is a method used to encourage the baby to turn.

Meconium – the earliest stool of a newborn baby. If it's present in the amniotic fluid, your baby may need additional monitoring and medical attention.

Precipitous labour – Describes a rapid labour. The potential risks include increased bleeding and the need for medical attention.

Postpartum haemorrhage (PPH) – this is heavy bleeding after birth, up to 12 weeks after having the baby. There are some factors that can increase your risk of PPH, though many women have no identifiable risk factors.

Retained placenta – when part or all of the placenta remains in the womb after birth, leading to potential complications.

Placental abruption – the separation of the placenta from the womb's wall before birth.

Abnormal heart rate of the baby – the variation of the baby's heart rate during labour.

Perinatal asphyxia – the lack of oxygen supply to the baby before birth.

Shoulder dystocia – where a baby's shoulder becomes stuck during birth.

PAIN RELIEF IN LABOUR

Relaxation methods – breathing techniques, massage, meditation and sound therapy can serve as distractions and promote relaxation during labour.

Aromatherapy – essential oils like clary sage, lavender and others can be used for their potential pain-relieving and calming effects. However, more research is needed to robustly recommend aromatherapy.

Water birth – the benefits of water birth include promoting endorphin release and providing comfort. Water birth can reduce the need for interventions like epidurals and shorten the first stage of labour.

Movement and position – adopting comfortable positions and using birthing tools like birthing balls and cushions can be helpful in the ease of your labour.

TENS machine – transcutaneous electrical nerve stimulation (TENS) is a method to release endorphins and disrupt pain signals.

Entonox (gas and air) – Entonox contains nitrous oxide and can be self-administered to reduce pain and anxiety, with no known side-effects on the baby.

Pethidine and diamorphine – these injections provide short-term pain relief but may cause drowsiness in the baby if administered too close to delivery.

Remifentanil – a patient-controlled pain relief method administered through a pump, with potential side-effects on the mother and baby.

Epidural – an injection into your back to provide anaesthesia to part of your body. Risks associated with it include prolonged labour and rare complications.

CHAPTER 6

POSTNATAL, BABY AND YOU

YOU'VE JUST GIVEN BIRTH. NOW WHAT?
BE PREPARED

It's natural to want to focus on the pregnancy and the labour whilst pregnant, but it can be helpful to know what to expect once you have given birth.

Your body has just undergone the most extraordinary feat, and even though you will be sore and feel bruised and battered, you probably won't notice it immediately after birth. You will only want to hear those first cries and be handed your beautiful baby. There are a few processes and hoops to jump through before you are left to your own devices. When you give birth, your midwife will first check your baby's APGAR (appearance, pulse, grimace, activity and respiration) score. It's such a quick assessment that you might not even notice it has been done, so do not worry. Providing all is well, you will be handed your baby for skin-to-skin contact within moments. The APGAR score goes up to 10, with a score of 7–10 indicating your newborn is in good health.

	2 points	1 point	0 points
Appearance – skin colour	Normal colour all over	Normal colour but hands and feet bluish	Blue all over
Pulse – heart rate	>100 beats per minute	<100 beats per minute	No pulse

	2 points	1 point	0 points
Grimace – reflexes	Grimaces, coughs, sneezes or pulls away when stimulated (usually a tube is placed in their nose)	Grimaces or cries weakly when stimulated	No reaction to being stimulated
Activity – muscle tone	Active movement	Some movement	No movement
Respiration – breathing rate and effort	Strong cry	Weak, slow or irregular breathing	No breathing

It is not often a baby scores a perfect 10, as quite commonly they have bluish hands and feet. I remember being surprised at how blue Harris' were. But this test will be done twice, usually at 1 minute and again at 5 minutes, and there is commonly an improvement in that time, often once the midwives have dried the baby with a towel or removed secretions from their airways and given them some oxygen. It is more likely your baby will score lower if they have been born prematurely, by Caesarean section, or if you had a complicated delivery. If the score is less than 5 at 1 minute, if it remains below 7 at 5 minutes, or if there is a specific problem like no pulse or no breathing, your baby will need special care to stabilise them. Only one in 100 full-term babies still have an APGAR score of less than 7 at 5 minutes[117].

SKIN-TO-SKIN CONTACT BE PREPARED

Skin-to-skin is simply the process of having your baby's bare skin in contact with and touching your bare skin, usually against your chest. This should be offered to you as soon after delivery as possible. Your little alien baby is covered in vernix (a white, creamy film that protects your baby's skin), blood and whatever other uterine debris you've ejected, but you won't care; you'll just want to hold it safely against yourself and probably cry. But there's so much more to this moment than just needing a good cuddle; skin-to-skin contact immediately after birth has some super-important health benefits for both you and your baby[118].

Benefits to you include an earlier delivery of the placenta, reduced bleeding, lower stress levels and improved confidence in breastfeeding your baby. Benefits to the baby include lower stress levels, less crying, regulating body temperature, improved breastfeeding initiation and optimal suckling.

You will notice there is so much more to it than the physiological advantages. This time of skin-to-skin after birth is almost magical. The scientist in me knows there is a biochemical reason for this, with your oxytocin 'love' hormone at a record high and your baby's catecholamine level (strengthening memory and learning) also peaking, but it feels so otherworldly and special.

Not to mention the SMELL. Your baby's head, as sticky and slimy as it is, will smell like heaven to you; this, again, is a chemical connection between you and your baby. But it is not just one way; your baby will also make this connection with the smell of your colostrum, and studies suggest that there is increased sensitivity to the odour of your milk the sooner after birth[119]. This early sensitivity and the high catecholamine levels that strengthen memory allow for a beautifully enhanced bond with your newborn baby.

Of course, not every mother will be able to have immediate skin-to-skin contact. Some babies may have to be taken for examination or treatment by the paediatrician, or some mothers will need to be examined or treated too. If that is the case, don't fret, it doesn't mean you and your baby won't bond. There will be plenty of time for your baby to feel, smell and touch you, and it is actually advised that you take the time to have skin-to-skin contact daily throughout the fourth trimester to help your baby feel safe and secure, and to aid brain development.

The art of snuggling does not need to be limited to just the mother; the father or other prominent figures in the baby's life can also partake in skin-to-skin contact. Whilst a lot of perinatal research focuses on the mother–baby bond, there have been some studies to look into the father–baby bond too. A review of these studies[120] showed that father–baby skin-to skin contact had positive impacts on both parties. The baby had improved temperature, pain and bio-physiological markers, and behavioural responses. The father had improved parental role attainment and interaction behaviour and reduced stress and anxiety. Therefore father–baby skin-to-skin contact should be promoted as a valuable alternative, especially if the mum is unavailable in the immediate postnatal period due to medical issues.

VITAMIN K BE PREPARED

Shortly after delivery, your baby will be offered a vitamin K injection. Vitamin K will help to prevent a rare bleeding disorder called haemorrhagic disease of the newborn, also known as vitamin K deficiency bleeding (VKDB), which can occur in the first few days of life. The main cause of this disease is vitamin K deficiency, which is an essential factor in blood clotting. This deficiency may occur because of certain drugs (for example, the antibiotic isoniazid used to treat TB, or medications to treat seizures, like phenytoin) that you have taken during pregnancy that may inhibit vitamin K, if there is not enough vitamin K in the breast milk (formula feeds are supplemented with vitamin K), or if the baby has a liver condition that does not allow the baby to absorb vitamin K from the feeds.

The injection is given in the baby's thigh and is only one dose. If you do not want your baby to have an injection, they can be offered oral doses, but they will need two doses in the first week and a further dose in one month (the timings of the doses can vary around the world). It is also worth knowing that it can taste bitter to the baby, so they may attempt to spit it out. Whilst the injection can cause pain and a small bruise at the injection site, it is considered more effective at preventing haemorrhagic disease of the newborn than the oral solution. This may be in part because of the staging of doses required, but also because there is no guarantee of how much is absorbed when babies frequently posset and vomit at this age.

Whilst vitamin K is highly recommended, remember that you can say no. Some parents are concerned by the lack of research that has gone into vitamin K. It is considered a very safe medication and has been given to millions of babies without concern worldwide, but more research could be done into potential side-effects and risks of vitamin K. It would also be helpful for us to understand better why babies are born with such low vitamin K levels in the first place.

If you decide to decline vitamin K, or are worried that the oral doses haven't been effective for your newborn, it is important to be vigilant for the signs and symptoms of the disease so they can be treated quickly. These are as follows:

- Blood in your baby's poo – this may look like fresh, bright red blood or thick, sticky black blood.
- Blood in your baby's urine.
- Bleeding from the nose, mouth or gums.
- Bleeding cord stump.
- Bruising.
- Tense fontanelle – this may feel like a bulging at the site of the fontanelle, often referred to as the 'soft spot' at the top of babies' heads.
- Pallor – skin looking paler than usual.

You can also always change your mind. If you have said no, but your baby is slow to feed or has some complications, which means they haven't fed as well as expected, their vitamin K level can be lower, so you may decide that you want to give them the treatment after all. Similarly, antibiotic treatment in yourself or your baby can also affect vitamin K levels, so you may want to change your mind and request the treatment, and that is totally acceptable.

CUTTING THE CORD BE PREPARED

The umbilical cord, which connects your baby to your placenta, offering a lifeline to the baby and supplying it with nutrients, is clamped and cut after birth. Neither you nor your baby can feel this process, which involves putting two clamps on the cord and using sterile scissors to cut between those two clamps. This is something your partner can request to do if you would like. There will be a stump left, which will eventually dry and fall off in the next couple of weeks. Traditionally, cord cutting was done immediately after birth as standard practice, but more recent evidence suggests this should be delayed.

DELAYED CLAMPING

Delayed cord clamping is defined differently around the world. The World Health Organisation (WHO) recommends waiting a minute before clamping[121]; the US, 30 to 60 seconds[122]; and the RCOG, 2 minutes[123]. Others might advise waiting until the cord has stopped pulsating before clamping it. An example supporting this might be that if the baby is lying above the height of the placenta for skin-to-skin, gravity is not on your side, so it may take longer for the blood to pump, and you may want to wait a couple of minutes longer; some literature advises up to 5 minutes[124].

Evidence suggests that babies can benefit from delaying the clamping process to allow the blood to transfer from the placenta to the baby fully. This can increase the amount of iron passed to the baby. Research shows that it increases haemoglobin at birth and improves the iron stores for the first 6 months of life.[125] Iron is needed for many functions, but certainly in the early months for neurodevelopment. It can also help to stabilise the baby, as there can be a sudden drop in blood pressure when they take their first breath in, due to movement of blood to the lungs, but this drop can be annulled by the excess blood transferred from the cord.

In terms of the risk of delayed cord clamping, it is considered safe and effective and the WHO recommends it, however, it has been suggested that it may increase the risk of neonatal jaundice and neonatal cardiopulmonary problems. On review, these studies suggesting adverse outcomes were mainly carried out in low- to moderate-income countries, and in a large, randomised control study carried out in a high-income country (Sweden) with full-term babies, they did not find an increase in the need of phototherapy for jaundice, or in the rate of respiratory symptoms. This suggests there may have been other confounding factors that increase these risks[126].

Where there might be a small increased risk of neonatal jaundice, it is usually mild, occurs commonly irrespective of delayed clamping, and can be treated simply with phototherapy, which is when the baby is placed under blue light.

Delayed clamping can't be performed in certain situations, for example, if you or the baby need immediate treatment and waiting for clamping would be inappropriate, or if the cord or placenta has a tear and needs to be clamped to prevent bleeding. Sometimes you can request the cord is 'milked' if you need the blood to be transferred more quickly, in order to offer treatment to you or your baby. It's a safe technique that simply involves pushing the blood through the cord more quickly. Delayed clamping is an absolute contraindication (which means that it is absolutely inadvisable, due to the risk of harm) in twins who share a placenta (monochorionic), as this could result in the movement of blood from one twin to the other, causing one to receive significantly more than the other.

You can have delayed cord clamping irrespective of whether you choose active or physiological management for the delivery of your placenta. You can also delay clamping with a Caesarean section.

MANAGING YOUR PERINEAL TEARS AND EPISIOTOMY BE PREPARED

Now we know the baby is safe and you're stable, it's time for *your* TLC. Your midwife will examine your perineum and vagina, and if you have any significant tears or have needed an episiotomy, you will require stitches, which they aim to do within an hour of giving birth. The degree of the tear determines the management. If you have had a first-degree tear, which is a small, skin-deep tear, you will usually be left alone to let it heal by itself. If you have had a second-degree tear that goes down to the muscle of the perineum, a third-degree tear that involves the anal sphincter muscle, or a fourth-degree tear that extends into the lining of the anus, you will be offered stitches.

This all sounds horrendous, and you imagine that the last thing you want is to be poked and prodded in an area already savaged, but in reality, with your babe in your arms, cooing at their every blink, you barely notice what's happening below. If you have had an epidural, you may not need further pain relief, but if you notice the sensation returning, you can ask for your epidural to be topped up. If you have not had an epidural, you will be given a local anaesthetic to numb the area first. They use dissolvable stitches, which will usually dissolve within a month.

I didn't notice my tears and the pain until two days later, when I felt like I had a red-hot poker up my bum. So, if you are in this less-than-fun poker situation, there are some ways to improve it:

Take painkillers – don't be a martyr. If you need pain relief, take it. Paracetamol and ibuprofen are safe to take postnatally, even if you are breastfeeding. Please do not take aspirin if you are breastfeeding. If you think you need stronger painkillers, your midwife or doctor can advise you which prescription medication is safe to take postnatally.

Use ice packs – Holly Willoughby recommended this to me! I was on *This Morning*, showing off my one-day-old baby via Skype, and I was in a postnatal euphoria. I had no issues with pain, felt on top of the world, and commented that I was 'Up and bouncing about.' Holly joked that she needed an ice pack down her pants for about a fortnight after she gave birth, so the following day, when it all started to kick in, the ice pack was the first thing I reached for. Cover the ice with a clean towel; do not place the ice directly onto your cuts.

Padsicles – you will need to wear pads after giving birth as you are likely to continue bleeding for up to 6 weeks. But you can give them a dual purpose by putting them in the freezer beforehand. The coolness helps to reduce the swelling and pain of both the perineal cuts and any haemorrhoids you may have developed. Some people even pimp up their padsicles by putting a bit of aloe vera on them before freezing, too.

The peri-bottle is your best friend – aside from your new baby, this device will be your most prized possession for the first couple of weeks. It's simple, just a bottle you can squirt water from. But don't be fooled; it is small but mighty. Whenever you pass urine, it can trickle over your cuts and stitches, which sting like hell, so the aim of the peri-bottle is to squirt warm water to dilute the urine and wash away the stinging wee. They have an upside-down design with an angled nozzle to make it easy for you to squeeze the water whilst on the loo. As well as neutralising the wee, they are really useful to help you clean so that you are not rubbing lots of abrasive tissue on your raw bits. Harris now plays with my peri-bottle in the bath as a squirting device, so it was well worth the purchase!

Do some wafting – let your vulva out. Take your pants off and waft it about in the fresh air for 10 minutes twice a day. When wearing pants, ensure they are not tight and are made from breathable fabrics.

Keep an eye out for infection – the pain usually lasts 2–3 weeks, but if it is horrible or lasts longer, there may be an infection. Signs of this can include hot, red and swollen skin, pus or discharge from the wound and a bad smell.

Poo with care – the softer your poo is, the easier it will be to pass without pain. Ensuring you drink plenty of fluids and eat a healthy diet high in fibre will help, but some new mums will also require laxatives. If you find the pressure of pooing hurts your cuts, you can press a clean pad or bunch of tissues on the wounds whilst you poo to help relieve the pressure. And, as always, remember to wipe from front to back to avoid the risk of infection. If you have haemorrhoids and are struggling to clean properly after a bowel motion, you may want to enlist your peri-bottle's help again.

THE FIRST FEED BE PREPARED

Babies are incredible. That little brown line that developed on your stomach (linea nigra), well, it's not just there to add another ugly pregnancy feature, nor are your darkening nipples. Both these changes were designed to help guide your poor-sighted newborn to your breasts. It's almost like a lit-up landing strip for the baby to see once it is born and for them to shimmy up and then find and latch onto the breast. In modern midwifery, we tend to just be handed our baby for skin-to-skin contact, so most babies don't necessarily have to do this shimmy. Still,

I distinctly remember Harris, who had temporarily been taken off me by the paramedics for checks, being placed back on my tummy rather than my chest, and him crawling his way up. These tiny, skinny arms and sharp fingernails were clawing their way up to my boobs like a zombie arm breaking through soil in a graveyard. It was an amazing effort for a being who couldn't even hold up his own head.

The baby will instinctively latch onto your nipple and start feeding, given the opportunity, so you can start the first feed as soon as you have been handed your newborn. If you have had a Caesarean section, and lying flat with a screen across your chest that is preventing you from being able to feed your baby, you may need to wait until you are in the recovery room and are more able to sit up in a comfortable and secure position to hold them.

They won't feed for long, as their stomachs are only the size of a marble at this point, so every drop of that colostrum milk is gold to them. They are, however, likely to want to feed regularly.

NEWBORN HEARING SCREEN BE PREPARED

If you have had a hospital birth, your baby may have its first newborn hearing screen prior to discharge. It is used to identify the one or two in 1,000 babies with hearing loss in one or both ears. Finding out early means earlier treatment, which gives babies a better chance of developing speech and language skills.

It involves putting a soft earpiece in the baby's ear, and then clicking sounds are played – this is known as an automated otoacoustic emission (AOAE). It only takes a few minutes and it does not harm your baby in any way. You will be given the results straight away.

In some cases second tests are required, as the first may be inconclusive if the baby was unsettled during the test, there was background noise, or the baby has fluid from the birth canal temporarily blocking the ear. This second test may be the same AOAE, or it may be a different test, called an automated auditory brainstem response (AABR). This involves placing sensors on your baby's head and then playing gentle clicking sounds through a pair of soft headphones. Again, this causes them no harm but it does take a little longer, between 5 and 15 minutes. If there is still no clear response from one or both ears, your baby will be referred to the audiologist for further investigation and management.

If the newborn hearing screen isn't done in the hospital, you will be given an appointment to do it within 3 weeks of birth.

FULL NEWBORN HEALTH CHECK BE PREPARED

If you have had a hospital birth, a healthcare professional specifically trained in the Newborn and Infant Physical Examination (NIPE) screening programme will usually carry out a full health check. This is likely to be the midwife or doctor in your postnatal ward. If you have had a home birth or you have been discharged before this examination could take place, you will be booked to have this done in the community (either at home or at a community clinic) within 72 hours of your baby's birth. This screening programme aims to identify and refer all children born with congenital abnormalities of the eyes, heart, hips and testes (in males) within 72 hours of birth.

At the NIPE screening, they will examine the following:

Eyes – the practitioner checks their position, symmetry and pupil size, looking to see if the baby maintains eye contact and the movement of the eyes. They will then shine a light in their eyes to look for signs of cataracts and test for a red reflex and a corneal light reflex. Around three or four in 10,000 babies have cataract problems needing treatment[127].

Heart – they will check the position of the heart, heart rate, rhythm and sounds, listening for any additional sounds like murmurs and checking on the femoral pulse volume. Around one in 100 babies has a heart problem[128].

Hips – they will check the symmetry of the hips and look at the skin folds for symmetry. They will also perform Barlow and Ortolani's manoeuvres, which test for developmental dysplasia of the hip. Around one or two in 1,000 babies have a hip problem needing treatment[129].

Testes – they will check testes in males to determine if they have descended. Around one in 100 boys have problems with the testes needing treatment[130].

Whilst the NIPE screening programme is designed to identify issues only in these four areas, other checks are often also performed, including the following:

Appearance – observing the colour of your baby, their breathing, posture, looking for any birthmarks or rashes, and listening to the sound of their cry.

Head – looking at their facial features and symmetry, examining the nose, mouth, ears and neck, feeling the fontanelles and examining their palate. A measurement of the head circumference will also be made.

Limbs – assessing the limbs, hands, feet and digits for completion, proportion and symmetry.

Lungs – observing the effort of breathing, noting the respiratory rate, and listening to the lung sounds.

Tummy – checking the tummy is soft and not causing pain, feeling the tummy for any masses and large organs, and ensuring the health of the umbilical cord.

Genitalia and anus – they will check for completeness and patency of genitalia and anus.

Spine – inspecting and feeling the spine's bones and checking the skin's integrity along the spine.

Movement, muscle tone and reflexes – examining the baby's tone, behaviour, movements, reflexes and posture primarily tests the central nervous system.

They will also ask you about your baby's bowel movements, urine, and how they are feeding and sleeping. The NIPE screening will be repeated at 6–8 weeks by your GP, so they can identify further any congenital abnormalities that can sometimes take time to become detectable.

Your baby must be naked for this examination, so if it takes place at home, ensure the room is warm enough to limit the discomfort to your baby. None of these procedures should hurt the baby, though it can feel uncomfortable being poked and prodded with cold implements and being out of your loving arms, so do not fear if there are some tears.

BIRTHMARKS BABY'S HERE

Birthmarks often worry parents, but they are widespread, and most do not require any form of treatment. Depending on the type of cell involved, there are several different types of birthmarks, mainly divided into pigmented or vascular birthmarks.

PIGMENTED BIRTHMARKS

Most pigmented birthmarks consist of cells containing the pigment melanin, which have all been collected together in one area to produce skin with a different colour. They can vary in size and are usually brown or black.

Mongolian blue spots – these are flat, bluish-grey birthmarks usually found on newborns' backs, buttocks or legs. They tend to be more common in babies with darker skin tones and usually fade by age four. They can look almost like big bruises and are often noted in your baby's records for safeguarding purposes. They are not signs of any underlying health condition, and no treatment is necessary.

Café-au-lait – these are light coffee-coloured marks that can be present at birth or develop soon after. A single spot is usually not a sign of anything significant. Still, more than six café-au-lait can indicate an underlying condition like neurofibromatosis type 1, so they will need to be investigated further.

Naevus of Ota – this is a mark on the face that appears blue, black or grey. They are more common in Asian populations. It typically affects one side of the face and may cause the eye to become discoloured, tending to remain throughout life, but it can be treated with a laser to lessen the appearance.

Congenital moles – these are similar to regular moles, but you are born with them rather than develop them. They are usually brown or black and can vary in size. It can increase the risk of developing skin cancer if they are particularly large.

VASCULAR BIRTHMARKS

Vascular birthmarks occur when blood vessels have not formed properly. They often look reddish or purplish.

Salmon patches/Angel kisses/Stork bites – these are common red or pink patches that are usually found on your baby's head, neck and eyelids, and tend to be more florid when they cry. Those on the eyelids and forehead tend to fade within 2 years, though others on the head and neck can persist for longer.

Haemangiomas – also known as strawberry marks, are raised, red or purplish marks that appear soon after birth. They are caused by an overgrowth of blood vessels that form a lump on the skin. They tend to get more prominent over the first 6 to 12 months but then usually shrink and disappear by age seven. If they obstruct the vision, breathing or feeding they may require medical treatment with medications such as propranolol or timolol.

Port wine stains – these are red, purple or dark patches, usually found on one side of the face and neck, though they can be found anywhere on the body. They are present at birth. There are two main treatments: laser treatment and cosmetic camouflage. Laser tends to make the birthmark lighter and is most effective on young children. Port wine stains that involve the upper part of the face can rarely be linked to underlying conditions, including Sturge-Weber syndrome, Klippel-Trenaunay syndrome and glaucoma.

We do not always know the exact cause of birthmarks, but many arise from genetic factors or vascular anomalies during early pregnancy when the blood vessels are forming. Birthmarks can mark your baby's individuality, and many parents grow to love this unique feature. The vast majority are harmless and do not need any intervention or treatment; however, if you have any concerns about your baby's birthmark, or it appears to be changing, is causing symptoms or interfering with essential functions, it is best to have them reviewed by a healthcare professional.

The red book

You will be given a red book, your child's health record, containing a record of your baby's height, weight, vaccinations and other important information. It should accompany you to all your child's midwife, health visitor and doctor appointments. It is a helpful guide to vaccination schedules, when to expect routine reviews and contains growth charts. Growth charts allow you to plot your baby's height and weight to see where they lie on average for their age. It is divided into centiles (which means out of 100), so if your child's height lies on the 50th centile, they are 'average', with 49 other children being shorter than them and 50 other children being taller. This growth chart is best used to track the individual's centile, so one would hope and expect your child to remain on or around the same centile over time, rather than using it as a comparison. If your child's height or weight starts dropping off, there may be concerns that they are not thriving as they should, and the doctor would want to investigate this. Though it should be noted that newborns are expected to lose weight initially, most babies will have returned to their birth weight by 3 weeks of age. If your baby loses more than 10 per cent of their birth weight or the weight doesn't return by 3 weeks, your midwife or doctor will assess them further[131].

CAESAREAN RECOVERY BE PREPARED

Whilst fairly safe and often straightforward, a CS is not the 'easy route', as some like to belittle it. It is major surgery. With this can come pain, nausea, fatigue and feelings of helplessness. The recovery process can vary from person to person, but a general guideline is that it will take up to 6 weeks. The average stay in hospital after a CS is around 2 to 4 days[132], though some go home sooner.

While in the hospital, you will be given pain relief and must stay in bed until all the anaesthetic has worn off, which can be a few hours. You will need help from the midwives and support workers with changing and feeding your baby. Once the anaesthetic has worn off, you will be encouraged to get out of bed and gently move around, as this will reduce your risk of blood clots, which is one of the risks of a CS, though you will need help to get out of bed and to lift your baby for at least the first day. You will keep the catheter in for at least 12 hours.

You may want nothing more than to rid yourself of your maternity wear, but after a CS the loose fitting around your tummy will offer relief from rubbing. In terms of pants, get as many hospital-issue disposable granny pants as you can.

Week 1: Inflammation – this is the initial stage of wound healing, where the body's immune response triggers inflammation at the CS site, leading to the typical redness, pain and swelling, and it may ooze a small amount of fluid. This process helps to clear away debris and start the healing process.

Weeks 2–3: Proliferation – during this stage, new blood vessels form and collagen (a protein that provides strength and structure) develops, marking the start of rebuilding damaged tissue. The incision may still look pink or red, but the wound edges might be starting to close.

Weeks 4–5: Remodelling – in this phase, the collagen fibres remodel to become more organised and aligned to improve the overall strength of the wound further. The scar is starting to become less noticeable.

Week 6: Recovery – as this stage implies, this period signifies ongoing recovery. You should be able to build up to and gradually resume most activities at this point. Your wound may still look reddish/purplish but it will gradually fade.

WHEN CAN I GO HOME? BE PREPARED

How soon you can go home depends on your and your baby's health, the kind of birth you had and where you had your baby. Some hospitals encourage early discharge, whereas others are more likely to hold on to you for a day or two.

If you had your baby in a maternity/birthing centre and all is well, you usually stay in the same room and can often go home between 6 and 12 hours after birth. If you need to stay for longer, you will probably be moved to a postnatal ward.

If you had your baby in a labour ward, you will get transferred to a postnatal ward after the delivery and can usually go home 6 to 12 hours later, providing there were no concerns. Before you are discharged, the midwives should have checked on your physical and mental health, that your placenta has been completely delivered, your perineum, that you have passed urine, signposted you to all the community care that is available for you and explained what to do if you are concerned by anything. They should also check that your baby has had a feed and opened their bowels. If you have any concerns about feeding, now is the time to voice them. Midwives should all be trained in basic support for feeding, be it bottle or breast, and you should be discharged feeling confident in either method. If you have had a home birth, the midwives usually stay for an hour to carry out the above checks and then you will be left at home.

If there are complications, you will be transferred to the high-dependency unit and then stepped down to a postnatal ward when you are stable. You may also need to stay longer if you had an emergency Caesarean section or your baby needs extra care. If your baby needs special care, they may be transferred to a neonatal unit. Different levels of care can be offered in neonatal units:

Special Care Baby Unit (SCBU) – this is a low-dependency unit for babies who do not need intensive care. Care usually includes monitoring their breathing and heart rate, giving them oxygen, keeping their body temperatures stable, treating low blood sugar and helping with feeds.

Local Neonatal Unit (LNU) – these babies may need a higher level of support. Usually, if a baby has been born below 32 weeks, they may be transferred here, where the care offered includes ventilation and breathing support, intensive care and feeding through a vein.

Neonatal Intensive Care Unit (NICU) – this offers babies the highest level of support. They may have been born before 28 weeks or were very unwell after birth. They may have severe disease affecting their breathing and need to be ventilated or require surgery.

Sometimes your baby still needs monitoring and treatment but is well enough to stay with you in a postnatal ward or a room in a neo-natal unit, which is called transitional care.

Whenever your discharge date is, remember that if you are travelling by car you will need a car seat to take your baby home, so buy this ahead of time, and make sure you know how to secure it.

YOUR FIRST 24 HOURS BE PREPARED

If, like me, you have a home birth or an uncomplicated vaginal delivery, your first 24 hours will likely be at home, without a midwife to fire a million questions at, which can feel daunting. If you have had to stay in the hospital overnight, you will usually be allowed to have one support person stay with you overnight and up to two visitors in the day, though some hospital policies may vary.

If your baby is well and can stay with you, you will have a bedside crib or a co-sleeper cot placed next to you. Hospitals are hot, light and noisy, so be prepared for your overnight stay with eye masks, appropri-ate clothing (for you and baby) and ear plugs (providing you can still hear your baby).

You may be visited by several different healthcare professionals and volunteers during your inpatient stay, including breastfeeding volunteers who may be able to help you with any feeding concerns, physiothera-pists to guide you through pelvic floor exercises and how to manage post-CS, nurses and midwives doing routine postnatal checks, and maternity support workers who will help support and look after you.

Depending on the journey to get to this point, people feel differ-ently. Some are exhausted, others exhilarated, but most likely you will experience a rollercoaster of both. Thankfully after those first couple of hours of alertness, many newborn babies get pretty sleepy, so all those horror stories about sleep, or lack of it, that you hear from zombified new parents don't necessarily apply to that first day. This is important, as you need to give yourself time to recover, so take this opportunity to sleep too. But your baby might have come out kicking and screaming and doesn't stop, and that can happen too; there is rarely a one size fits all, but check they aren't hungry, tired, hot or cold. It might feel like a total guessing game, but eventually you will understand your baby's cues and what each screech, whimper and moan means. Either way, your baby will likely need to feed every 2–3 hours, so even if they are having a wonderful snooze, the advice is to wake the baby up so that they are getting at least eight feeds in 24 hours. Again, this is just a guideline; my boobmonster would wake every 40 minutes to an hour for feeds in those early days.

Your baby will likely pass its first meconium (poo) on this first day. As previously discussed, this can sometimes occur when the baby is still in the amniotic sac, but this is the exception, not the rule. So it is probable that on this first day you will see black, tarry and sticky poo in their nappy. This type of poo is made up of skin cells, hair, amniotic fluid and other debris swallowed by your baby whilst they were in your womb. The colour and consistency will change over the next few days as they start to feed more. If you are breastfeeding, it tends to be runnier and mustard-coloured, and if you are bottle feeding, it can be a little firmer and pale brown or yellow-green. If your baby hasn't passed meconium in the first 24 hours, inform your midwife, as this will need to be monitored. Your baby should also pass urine in the first 24 hours, though it can be difficult to know if this has happened if the amount produced is tiny or if it has happened at the same time as the bowels opening. Once feeding has been established by days three to four, your baby will have more frequently wet nappies.

If you feel overwhelmed on night one, cut yourself some slack. You might have seen your midwife swaddle your baby like a burrito in a matter of seconds, and it will take you 20 minutes. Or you saw them getting your baby dressed in a babygrow so swiftly, but you're there with your screaming newborn who is cold and annoyed at you, but you just can't figure out how the little button snaps line up. That is ok. It's a huge learning curve; it will be slow, and mistakes will be made, but each one gives you experience and knowledge. Your hormones will be all over the place, and you will be recovering from a huge physical event that has caused you exhaustion and pain, so approach yourself with the same kindness, grace and love that you will show your new baby. You don't have to be perfect; you just need to be safe and survive.

BLEEDING AFTER BIRTH BE PREPARED

In addition to all these joys, you also have lochia (postpartum bleeding) to look forward to. All women will bleed after birth, irrespective of whether they had a vaginal or Caesarean birth. This is a mixture of blood, mucus and tissue from the womb, a bit like a menstrual period. It usually lasts up to 6 weeks, but in some women it can last longer, up to 12 weeks. It tends to start off quite heavy with bright red or brownish blood, but as the weeks progress it becomes lighter in both volume and colour. As it can be quite heavy initially, you will want to have enough pads to hand (avoid tampons until after your 6-week check, due to the increased risk of infection). It can be even heavier at the start if you are breastfeeding as the oxytocin released from breastfeeding causes increased contractions of your womb, though overall the same amount of blood is lost as if you are not breastfeeding. Maternity pads are a bit more absorbent and heavy-duty than regular sanitary pads, especially for the first week when it is heavy and can contain larger clots. I also wore disposable pants, as the thought of having to stand over a sink washing blood out of my knickers with one hand whilst nursing a baby in the other is really not cool. Whilst blood clots are common initially, passing a lot of large clots in the first 24 hours can be a sign of a postpartum haemorrhage and should be flagged up with a healthcare professional immediately. You can still also get secondary postpartum haemorrhage between 24 hours and 12 weeks, often associated with an infection, so your bleeding becoming heavier rather than lighter is another sign to look out for.

Nappies

It is worth going through nappy options to make sure you are stocked up with the right stuff for your first few weeks. The nappy sizes depend on the weight of your baby, which, of course, you will not know until you meet said baby. So, unless you have been told beforehand, based on scans, that your baby is particularly big or small, I would suggest buying small packs of both size 0 and size 1 nappies in preparation. If you leave them unopened and hold on to the receipts, you can always return the unused pack. Size 0 nappies are for low birthweight or premature babies, and size 1 tends to be for your 'normal' full-term newborns. At this stage, you can ignore all the 'active fit' and 'pull up' options as they are aimed at the more mobile, older ages. Our priority now is to keep the baby dry and the excrement contained! The exact weights might differ from brand to brand, but the general rule of thumb is as follows:

- Size 0 (1–2.5kg, 2–5lbs)
- Size 1 (2–5kg, 5–11lbs)
- Size 2 (3–6kg, 7–14lbs)
- Size 3 (4–9kg, 8–20lbs)
- Size 4 (7–18kg, 15–40lbs)
- Size 5 (11–25kg, 24–55lbs)
- Size 6 (16kg+, 35lbs+)

Though, to be honest, I never recall basing which size we went for on Harris' weight. We usually just upped the size when the tapes felt a bit stretched, if there were any obvious marks from the nappies on his legs, or if they started leaking more, which usually indicated it was not absorbent enough. Once you are confident in the sizing, buy in bulk, as the average newborn will go through 310 nappies in the first month! We also tended to opt for the cheaper brands by day, when we would be changing the nappy more often, and the more expensive (and hopefully more absorbent!) brands in the night to limit 3am costume changes. But one size does not fit all, and some babies' beautiful rumps suit certain brands, so if you are not succeeding on the containment front, try other brands.

COMMUNITY MIDWIFE VISITS BE PREPARED

Wherever you had your baby, you will not be left to your own devices for too long at home. The community midwife will be scheduled to visit you the day after discharge, and the midwifery care will continue for usually 10 days after the birth of your baby, after which you will be discharged into the care of your Health Visitor and GP. In some cases where parents need additional support, the midwives can continue their care for up to 28 days. The initial visit is usually done at home, but subsequent ones can be at local venues like children's centres and health centres. There is no set number of visits you will be booked in for, but most mothers are seen at least three times. During these visits, the midwife will assess your baby for signs of jaundice, infection of the umbilical cord or eyes, and thrush in the mouth. If you are breast-feeding, your baby will be weighed on day three. You will also have a visit booked for day five, for the blood spot test.

BLOOD SPOT TEST

The blood spot test (also known as a heel prick test) is performed when your baby is ideally 5 days old but can be done up to day eight. It involves pricking your baby's heel and getting four drops of blood onto a card. It shouldn't cause too much distress, but keeping them warm, comfortable and in your arms will help. I fed Harris throughout this test, and he didn't even flinch.

This tests for nine different rare but serious conditions:

Sickle cell disease – this is a genetic blood disorder in which the haemoglobin in the red blood cells forms abnormally. Haemoglobin is a protein that carries oxygen from the lungs to various parts of the body. The abnormal haemoglobin causes the red blood cells to become rigid and take on a crescent or 'sickle' shape instead of their usual round shape, making the blood cells more fragile, and they tend to get stuck in small blood vessels. This can lead to a decreased ability to carry oxygen and cause a blockage of blood flow.

Cystic fibrosis – this is a genetic disorder that primarily affects the respiratory and digestive systems. It is caused by mutations in a gene, which leads to the production of a faulty protein. This defective protein disrupts the normal flow of salt and water in and out of cells, resulting in the production of a thick, sticky mucus that can clog airways and various organs in the body.

Congenital hypothyroidism – this is a condition in which a baby is born with an underactive thyroid gland or the thyroid gland is absent. The thyroid gland produces thyroid hormones that play a crucial role in regulating metabolism and the body's energy levels, which is essential for healthy growth and development, particularly of the brain and nervous system.

Phenylketonuria (PKU) – this is a genetic disorder in which a deficiency or absence of an enzyme called phenylalanine hydroxylase inhibits the body's inability to properly process an amino acid called phenylalanine. Amino acids are the building blocks of proteins, and phenylalanine is obtained from the diet, especially from high-protein foods. As a result, phenylalanine levels in the blood become abnormally high, which can lead to several complications that particularly affect brain development and function.

Medium-chain acyl-CoA dehydrogenase deficiency (MCADD) – this is a genetic disorder that affects the body's ability to break down certain types of fats (medium-chain fatty acids). MCADD is caused by mutations in the gene, which encodes an enzyme essential for the breakdown of medium-chain fatty acids into usable energy during periods of fasting or increased energy demands. This leads to an accumulation of fatty acid metabolites and a deficiency of energy production.

Maple syrup urine disease (MSUD) – this is a genetic disorder that affects the body's ability to break down certain amino acids found in proteins. In MSUD, the enzymes needed for this breakdown are deficient or nonfunctional, leading to an accumulation of the amino acids and their toxic byproducts in the blood and tissues. It is named after the sweet smell of the affected individual's urine, similar to the scent of maple syrup.

Isovaleric acidaemia (IVA) – this is a genetic disorder caused by a deficiency of an enzyme needed for the breakdown of the amino acid leucine. This leads to the accumulation of toxic metabolites in the blood and tissues.

Glutaric aciduria type 1 (GA1) – this is a genetic disorder caused by a deficiency of the enzyme crucial for the breakdown of certain amino acids, leading to the accumulation of toxic substances in the blood and tissues. These substances can damage the brain and nervous system, particularly the basal ganglia, which are important for coordinating movement.

Homocystinuria (pyridoxine unresponsive) (HCU) – this genetic disorder is caused by deficiencies in the enzymes or cofactors involved in the breakdown of homocysteine, a certain amino acid, resulting in its accumulation in the blood and tissues.

CORD CARE

During your visits, your midwife will check your baby's cord to ensure it is healthy, drying up normally, and make sure there are no signs of an infection. You will also be shown how to look after the cord area. The cord will usually dry up and fall off within 1 and 3 weeks of cutting and clamping, and the clip (used to clamp it) is left on and will fall off along with the cord. In the interim, you need to keep the area clean and dry. It is also helpful to fold the baby's nappy down at the front so that the cord and clip are exposed rather than covered by the nappy. You should also look out for signs of infection, which include redness around the skin on the tummy, and the cord itself becoming sticky or smelly.

JAUNDICE BE PREPARED

Jaundice is a yellow discolouration of the skin and eyes, secondary to the build-up of a chemical called bilirubin, which results from the breakdown of the baby's red blood cells. It is a normal process and doesn't mean the baby is unwell. It usually appears on day three or four and goes by about day 10, though it can last longer in breastfed babies. However, it can sometimes be associated with other conditions, especially if it occurs within 24 hours of the baby's birth or lasts for over 3 weeks. If the doctor or midwife suspects an abnormally high level of jaundice, they are likely to take a blood test to determine if they need phototherapy – a light therapy – to reduce it.

You can judge me for this, but I thought my baby boy came out with wonderfully olive and tanned skin. I was secretly smug that he had inherited my genes over his father's, who is significantly paler and frecklier. However, when Harris was a couple of months old, I took him to meet some friends, who were all doctors, and one of them, who was a paediatrician, started asking me some questions about Harris' health. Usually, when friends meet your brand-new baby, they just coo and aah and tell you how adorable they are (even if they do just look like a roast chicken), but he was asking me about his stool, feeding, urine, etc. So I cut to the chase and asked him what he was getting at, to which he responded that he thought Harris had jaundice and that I should probably get it checked out! Fast-forward to a rapid access paediatric clinic and, yes, it was confirmed he had jaundice; it was mild and under the threshold for treatment, but, alas, it meant his gloriously golden tinge was actually just a whole load of bilirubin that, in time, faded to reveal his father's alabaster skin!

THE FOURTH TRIMESTER   BE PREPARED

I am a doctor, and I am ashamed to say I hadn't heard of the fourth trimester until I had my own baby. This is the time of adjustment in the first 12 weeks after having your baby, and it is as important as the three trimesters preceding it for both mother and baby's health. This transitional period can be a useful concept for parents as a reminder that your baby will probably cry a lot, it will be hard, but it's not forever. Your newborn has been launched into a cold, bright, loud environment, and has to cry for sleep, food, nappy changes, warmth and love. Until this point, they have been entirely cocooned, sleeping when they want to, being fed constantly, and feeling warm and secure, so these 12 weeks will serve as a time to allow your baby to adjust to this brand-new world. Whilst, of course, not all babies adjust in this exact timeframe, it is helpful to be given a guideline and a goal to work towards as a sleep-deprived parent! Whilst your baby is trying to adjust to the new world, you are also adjusting to life as a parent. Whether motherhood is something you have dreamt of for years or if it is something that was somewhat sprung on you, this period unifies everyone and is difficult for everyone alike. It can feel reassuring to know that new parents worldwide are having the same wobbles, fears and moments of 'Why did I do this again!? Send him back!'

YOUR 6–8-WEEK POSTNATAL CHECK
BABY'S HERE

You should book a 6–8-week postnatal check with your GP to ensure you recover well after the birth. Many practices will arrange this to be done on the same day as your baby's 6–8-week baby check, as managing to leave the house for one appointment is stressful enough, but if it's easier for you to have them on separate days, or you (quite rightly) want to focus on just yourself at this appointment, do ask.

Baby brain may not be a medical term, but it is a thing. Your cerebral ventricles have turned into mashed-up bananas, so I always recommend you write a list of all your questions or concerns before your appointment so that the standard doctor's surgery amnesia doesn't hit. The GP will allow you to discuss your birth experience at the appointment. They may cover the following issues:

- Symptoms and signs of postnatal mental health problems (see postnatal depression, page 154).
- Symptoms and signs of postnatal physical problems including:
    - infection
    - pain
    - vaginal discharge and bleeding
    - bladder function
    - bowel function
    - nipple and breast discomfort – your GP may examine your breasts if you are having any breast pain. You may be referred on for feeding support if needed.
- Blood clots – your GP will ask about any swelling, tenderness, or redness to your legs that could indicate a blood clot.

- Anaemia – it is normal to feel tired when you have a new baby, but if your fatigue is out of keeping with what is expected, it may be a sign of anaemia. As can be shortness of breath, pallor, dizziness and palpitations.
- Preeclampsia/gestational hypertension – your GP will check your blood pressure (and possibly urine) if you developed preeclampsia or gestational hypertension during pregnancy.
- The importance of pelvic floor exercises and a reminder of how to do them.
- Perineal healing, if you have had a vaginal birth – if you had an episiotomy or required stitches, your GP might offer to examine it to ensure it is healing well.
- Wound healing – if you have had a Caesarean section your GP will offer to examine the wound.
- Your GP may examine your tummy to ensure the womb has shrunk back down into the right position and that there is no pain or tenderness.
- Lifestyle factors, including diet, physical activity, smoking, alcohol and drug use.
- Contraception and sex.
- Safeguarding concerns.
- Signposting to birth support and birth reflection services.
- Smear tests – if your cervical screening was due whilst you were pregnant, it can be booked in for 12 weeks postnatally.

POSTNATAL DEPRESSION BABY'S HERE

Postnatal depression (PND) and baby blues are two common emotional conditions that can affect new mothers (and fathers) after giving birth, but they differ in severity, duration and symptoms.

Baby blues is a mild and short-lived condition that affects up to 80 per cent of new mothers[133]. It typically develops within a few days of giving birth and lasts up to 2 weeks. Some symptoms of baby blues include mood swings, anxiety, sadness, irritability and crying spells.

These symptoms are usually mild and do not interfere with the mother's ability to care for herself or her baby. I remember at one point watching Harris sleeping peacefully and suddenly bursting into uncontrollable tears when I realised that one day he would love someone more than me! My only morsel of advice during this hormonal stage is to wear sunglasses if you don't want everyone at the supermarket, station, pharmacy and park to offer you a sad consolatory look and a warm hand on the shoulder. The tears came thick and fast, like a broken faucet, without an obvious trigger, but as quickly as they were turned on, they just suddenly stopped one day. Baby blues is a common and expected postnatal stage, and it is helpful to normalise it by discussing it openly and reaching out to your partner, family and friends, or other parents going through the same thing, for a quick support boost.

Postnatal depression, on the other hand, is a more severe and longer-lasting condition that can develop within weeks or months after giving birth. It affects about 10 per cent of new mothers[134] and can last several months or even longer if left untreated. Symptoms of postnatal depression are similar to those of baby blues but are more intense and persistent. These symptoms can interfere with the mother's ability to care for herself and her baby. They may include feelings of sadness, hopelessness, guilt, loss of interest in activities, changes in appetite and sleep patterns, and thoughts of self-harm or harming the baby.

Postnatal depression is a treatable condition, and the approach may vary depending on the severity of your symptoms and individual needs. Help is out there in many forms, including but not limited to the following:

Lifestyle changes – regular exercise, eating a healthy diet, getting enough sleep and reducing stress. Honestly, I say all these things a little tongue-in-cheek. 'Getting enough sleep and reducing stress' is almost laughable in the newborn stage, and as for exercise, does walking around the kitchen island 4,000 times at 3am repeating the phrase 'good boy' and trying to get your insomniac infant to sleep count? I suppose it is just a matter of doing what you can to help yourself, but know that subsequent treatments come into play.

Support groups and talking – friendship and family groups are often essential outlets for new mums (see find your crew, page 175); however, these might not be an option for some. Joining a support group for new mothers can help provide social help and alleviate feelings of isolation and loneliness outside the traditional emotional support network. MumsAid is a perfect example of one such charity in the UK, which offers a great way to talk with others going through many of the same challenges.

Mindfulness techniques – mindfulness-based therapies can help reduce symptoms of depression by promoting relaxation and self-awareness. You probably won't have many spare hours to read books on it, but there are loads of apps to help guide you through mindfulness and meditation that you can listen to whilst you feed, or do the washing, etc. Personally I use the app Headspace, which has guided me through numerous mindful exercises, and has also helped me get back to sleep when anxious thoughts infiltrate my mind. I have also used the Calm app, which has the added bonus of hearing Matthew McConaughey's dulcet tones as he reads you a bedtime story. His Southern voice, dripping with charm, is worth the listen even if you have no issues falling asleep, and if anyone is going to help you 'ponder the depth of the present moment', it's him.

Medication – antidepressant medication may be prescribed to help relieve the symptoms of postnatal depression. Selective serotonin reuptake inhibitors (SSRIs) are commonly prescribed for postnatal depression, and they are generally considered safe for breastfeeding mothers, though this should be discussed with your healthcare provider.

Therapy – cognitive-behavioural therapy (CBT) is a talking therapy that helps mothers identify and change negative thought patterns and behaviours contributing to depression. Interpersonal therapy (IPT) is another therapy that focuses on improving relationships and social support.

Traumatic births can be a trigger for postnatal depression. A traumatic experience varies from person to person but may include elements of extreme pain, complications, emergency medical interventions, feelings of loss of control or fear for your baby's health. Where these experiences have lasting emotional impact, they can lead to postnatal depression or other mental health conditions like post-traumatic stress disorder. It is important to acknowledge and validate your feelings about your traumatic birth experience, allowing yourself to be angry, grieve, or cry. You do not have to minimise your emotions for the sake of anyone else.

Some hospital trusts offer a birth debriefing session, which I encourage you to attend. During this session, you can discuss your experience, usually with a midwife who has reviewed your case, who will let you express your emotions and help provide some clarity and hopefully some closure. These sessions can occur soon after the birth, but can also be requested years later, and should you need further support following on from this session, this can also be arranged.

If your hospital trust does not offer a debriefing session you can access psychological support directly via your GP, who can refer you to a perinatal mental health team or for talking therapies, and some areas allow for self-referral. There are also a number of support groups including the Birth Trauma Association and the Traumatic Support Group at BabyCentre.

Postpartum psychosis

While many people may experience the 'baby blues' and some suffer from postnatal depression, around one in 500 mothers can experience postpartum psychosis within hours or days after giving birth. This is a very serious mental illness, and you should contact your GP immediately if you think a mother is experiencing any symptoms, or go to A&E or call 999 if you think mother, baby or any other connected person might be in danger of harm.

Common symptoms include:

- Hallucinations
- Delusional thoughts
- Mania – 'high' episodes, talking quickly or racing thoughts, feeling restless

- Depression or low mood – tearful, lacking energy, loss of appetite, anxiety, sleep deprivation
- Combination of alternating mania and depression
- Loss of inhibitions and behaving oddly
- Feeling suspicious, anxious, confused

Postpartum psychosis is treatable but it usually requires hospitalisation, where the condition can be treated with prescription medication, electroconvulsive therapy or cognitive behavioural therapy (CBT).

SEX AND CONTRACEPTION BABY'S HERE

You may be thinking that sex is the last thing on your mind after you've just given birth. And you're probably right, at the beginning, when you're still sore, knackered and you have a baby in the room with you at all times, it may be a distant thought. But at some point you may want to have sex again, and at that point the likelihood is that you don't want to get pregnant again straight away. Hence the Faculty of Sexual and Reproductive Healthcare (FSRH) recommends that breastfeeding and non-breastfeeding mothers commence effective contraception as soon as possible after delivery[135]. This allows new mothers to plan any subsequent pregnancy and avoid short interpregnancy intervals, as an interval of less than 12 months between having your baby and conceiving again is associated with an increased risk of complications like premature delivery, low birth weight and small for gestational age babies.

Your GP should discuss contraception with you at your 6–8-week check, but don't be afraid to bring it up if they don't. Return of fertility can vary significantly, but the earliest known time of ovulation is 27 days after delivery, so no contraception is needed for the first 21 days, but this is still before the 6–8-week check, so do speak to your GP or a Sexual Health Clinic sooner if you are planning to have sex before this appointment.

WHEN IS THE RIGHT TIME TO HAVE SEX AGAIN?

This is entirely a personal choice; you can start having sex again whenever you feel physically and emotionally ready. On average, 89 per cent of women resume sex within 6 months of giving birth, but we also know that sexual dysfunction rates vary from 41–83 per cent at 2–3 months postpartum, to 64 per cent at 6 months[136]. Some studies suggest that even after 18 months postpartum women still have markedly lower levels of sexual pleasure[137]. It's worth noting that pre-pregnancy sex isn't perfect either, with rates of sexual dysfunction running at around 38 per cent[138]. Ultimately, postpartum lack of libido is a normal experience for many women, but it is usually temporary. So communicate with your partner and/or with your doctor, and know that with time, patience and communication, you are likely to regain sexual enjoyment soon enough.

WHY MIGHT YOU HAVE A LOW SEX DRIVE POSTNATALLY?

- Hormones – your body has gone through extreme hormonal changes, and a reduction in oestrogen and progesterone can impact sexual desire and arousal.
- Discomfort – following on from delivery, you may still be feeling sore, and having sex can be uncomfortable, making the thought of it unappealing.
- Body confidence – your body has changed, and you may not be comfortable in your own skin yet. Feeling self-conscious, having a negative body image and low self-esteem can all decrease sexual desire.
- Fatigue – newborns are exhausting, and when you are sleep-deprived and physically on your knees, having the libido for sex may not be a priority.
- Mental health – the stress and anxiety of caring for a newborn can reduce your sex drive. If you are suffering from postnatal depression, this may have an even more profound effect on your libido.
- Breastfeeding – prolactin, a hormone produced during breastfeeding, suppresses the production of oestrogen and progesterone, reducing sexual desire and arousal and causing vaginal dryness. Even just the physical and emotional demands of breastfeeding might be enough to put you off sex for a while.

WHAT ARE YOUR CONTRACEPTIVE OPTIONS?

The choices can depend on whether you are breastfeeding and how early you would like to start the contraception. Follow the flowchart below to see your options:

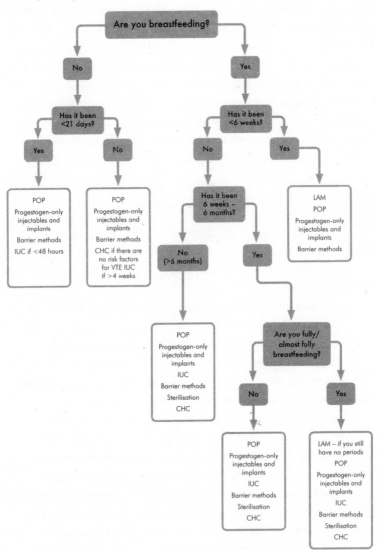

Progestogen-only pill (POP) – this is often referred to as 'the mini pill'. You will note from the flowchart that it is offered to ALL women after giving birth (unless they have a medical reason that they cannot use it), as it is incredibly safe. The POP can be started immediately after delivery without the need for any additional contraceptive precautions. If it is started after day 21, you must ensure you are not already pregnant and additional contraception is needed for 2 days after taking your first pill.

Progestogen-only injectables and implants – like the POP, these are considered very safe forms of contraception and can also be offered to all women immediately after birth.

Lactational amenorrhoea (LAM) – fully breastfeeding women (those doing at least 4-hourly feeds in the day and 6-hourly feeds at night) can rely on lactational amenorrhoea for contraception for the first 6 months after delivery so long as they haven't had a period. This method relies on a postpartum woman's natural infertility associated with breastfeeding. A baby's suckling causes a reduction in gonadotropins, which suppresses ovulation and is 98 per cent effective[139]. If the woman reduces her breastfeeding, has a period, or is past the 6-month postpartum mark, there is a loss in the contraceptive effect, and it is no longer recommended as an effective form of contraception. To reiterate, the LAM method is only 98 per cent effective if all of the following applies:

- Your baby is under six months old.
- You are breastfeeding at least 4-hourly in the day.
- You are feeding at least 6-hourly at night.
- You are not having periods.
- Your baby has not started eating food or drinking other liquids.

Combined Hormonal Contraception (CHC) – this form of contraception has both progesterone and oestrogen in it and includes the combined oral contraceptive pill, the patch and the vaginal ring. Oestrogen can increase your risk of blood clots, and in the first few weeks postpartum you are at your highest risk, but after 21 days this risk is reversed and CHC can be used. Previously it had been advised that women who were breastfeeding should not be given the CHC under 6 months after birth due to concerns of the oestrogen transferring to the baby and affecting their growth; however, this has not been proven, and in 2016, the guidelines were changed to allow for the use of CHC after 21 days even in breastfeeding mothers[140].

Intrauterine contraception – this is known to most as 'the coil', and it includes both the intrauterine system (IUS), which contains progesterone, and the intrauterine device (IUD), which contains copper. Immediate insertion (within 48 hours of childbirth) performed by a specifically trained clinician is considered a safe, effective and convenient form of contraception, and it is associated with high continuation rates. Outside of those 48 hours, it is not advised to be inserted until 28 days after childbirth because the risk of perforating the womb is increased, especially if the mother is breastfeeding, and because the risk of expelling the coil is also higher.

Barrier methods – this includes both female and male condoms and can be used immediately. If you would like to use a diaphragm or cap, please note they are 92–96 per cent effective if used correctly[141], and can only be used from around 6 weeks after giving birth.

Sterilisation – female sterilisation is an operation to block or seal the fallopian tubes, preventing the eggs from becoming fertilised, and is a safe option for permanent contraception after childbirth. It is highly effective (>99 per cent)[142], however, it is essential to know that some long-acting contraceptive methods (like the coil, the implant, the injection, etc.) are as, or more, effective than female sterilisation. Whilst it can be carried out immediately after birth, ideally, it should be performed after some time has elapsed, to reduce the risk of possible regret. The failure rate of sterilisation (<5/1,000 women) is the same whether it was performed immediately after birth or after an interval. Due to this risk of regret, sterilisation is not performed at the same time as a Caesarean section unless counselling has taken place and the decision is made at a time separate (at least 2 weeks in advance) from a planned Caesarean section.

YOUR POSTNATAL BODY BABY'S HERE

'Bouncing back' is up there with ' is it that time of the month?' in one of the worst phrases to happen to women. The media dissects the bodies of celebrities who have just given birth, and congratulates them on returning to their former physical glory, but no one focuses on the need to rest and recover; no one really cares about what is happening to their body and mind behind the external image.

Dieting or exercising too soon after being pregnant and giving birth not only has an effect on your mental health at a time when you are often already feeling your most vulnerable, but it can result in a prolapse, urinary incontinence, excessive bleeding and reduced milk supply. So let us normalise the postnatal body and what to expect from it.

YOU WILL STILL LOOK PREGNANT

This tends to be a shock for first-time mums. Yes, your baby is out, but your womb still needs time to shrink back down, you still need to lose retained fluid, and your stomach muscles still need to come back together. All these factors make for a body that still looks 6 months pregnant in the first 6 to 8 weeks, or longer in some. Please think twice before buying compression belts (also called postnatal shapewear or belly wraps) for your stomach after birth. There are some medical-grade postpartum girdles that your healthcare provider may advise to offer support, but note there is no evidence that they will 'shrink your belly', help you to lose weight or reshape your stomach or hips; in fact, in some cases, they may even make prolapse worse.

YOUR HIPS WILL BE WIDER

I was surprised when I tried to put on a cute little denim pinafore dress 6 months after I had Harris, and it just wouldn't zip around my hips. This is because during pregnancy, due to the role of the hormone relaxin loosening up the ligaments that hold the pelvis together, the pelvis tilts and becomes, on average, around 2.5cm wider. For most, this will come back together again, but, in some cases, it doesn't always go back to how it was even if you are back to your pre-pregnancy weight. Interestingly, the same can happen with your rib cage, with it becoming wider to accommodate for your growing womb, and it may or may not shrink back to your pre-pregnancy width.

YOUR CAESAREAN SECTION HEALING WILL TAKE LONGER THAN YOU THINK

Women are often advised that they can take up to 6–8 weeks to heal and at that mark they are back to lifting, driving and life as normal. However, underneath that (hopefully) beautifully healed scar, at 6 weeks the abdominal fascia, which holds organs and muscles in place, has regained less than 60 per cent of its original strength[143]. It can take over 5 months to reach the 100 per cent tensile strength mark. So, although you may look in the mirror and think you are back on track, progress slowly and steadily to avoid injury.

YOU MAY HAVE DARKER BITS OF SKIN

The linea nigra is a dark vertical line that runs down the middle of the abdomen and it appears in 90 per cent of pregnant women, usually in the first trimester. It is caused by the increased production of melanin due to the effects of oestrogen and progesterone. It tends to be more prominent in those with darker complexions, and it can increase in width and intensity as the pregnancy progresses. It usually fades gradually after delivery, but in some women it can persist. In my case the line above my belly button disappeared and the line below it persisted, although it did fade considerably. Medical treatment is not necessary, but if you are unhappy with it cosmetically, try to avoid sun exposure as this can make it become darker and more obvious. There is also some evidence that folic acid can reduce the formation of linea nigra[144]. We are all advised to take this in supplementation form in the first 12 weeks of pregnancy anyway, but thereafter you can consider whether you are getting enough of this vitamin in your diet (through leafy green vegetables, citrus fruits, legumes, fortified cereals). Bleaching creams have also been used, though the results have not always been satisfactory, and note these cannot be used during pregnancy or breastfeeding. It is not only on your stomach that you may notice increased pigmentation; your areolas will darken to help your baby see where to latch (see page 193), and some women also develop melasma, which are patches of more pigmented skin on the face. Again, these are likely to fade within a few months of delivery, but some may not.

YOU MAY HAVE A DIASTASIS RECTI

This is the separating of the two muscles (recti muscles) that run down the middle of the stomach. The two halves of the muscles are attached in the middle by a connective tissue called the linea alba. In pregnancy, the womb pushes apart the muscles to make room for the growing baby and the linea alba thins. The muscles usually go back together by 8 weeks postnatally, however, some can take longer and may need the help of physiotherapy. The degree of separation can vary, and in some it can appear like a long bulge in the middle of your stomach, whereas in others it may not be at all visible, or only cones or domes (bulges) when you contract your stomach muscles. You can test to see if you have a diastasis recti by lying on your back with your legs bent, then slightly lifting your head and shoulders off the floor. Feel the midline of your stomach and place your fingers in the gap between the recti abdominis muscles above and below your belly button. If you can fit two or more fingers in the gap it is likely you have a diastasis recti. You should expect the number of fingers you can fit in this gap to gradually reduce in the postnatal period. If it does not, do seek care, even if it is not bothering you aesthetically, as it can result in back pain in the long term.

YOU MAY NOTICE STRETCH MARKS

These are the lines that develop on the skin where it has been stretched by pregnancy, often around the stomach, but this can happen in other areas, including the hips, breasts and thighs. They tend to start developing around the end of the second trimester and, depending on your skin tone, can look pink, purple, red or brown. Most women will develop some, though the extent can vary from mother to mother. Rapid weight gain in pregnancy can be a contributing factor, but mostly it is down to your skin elasticity. Good lifestyle habits like a healthy diet and exercising can have a role in skin elasticity, but is largely down to your genetics. Stretch marks are a natural and expected part of pregnancy, but whilst some mothers will view them as their stripes of honour, others will feel more self-conscious about them. Whilst there are no high-quality studies to suggest any lotion or potion will prevent stretch marks, we do know that emollients (moisturisers and oils) keep the skin hydrated and thus can help to promote wound healing and skin repair. Eventually your stretch marks will start to fade on their own and they tend to turn a less noticeable pale or silvery colour. Some treatments, including retinol creams, laser, microneedling and chemical peels, can be used to lessen the appearance, though these should not be used whilst pregnant, and some cannot be used whilst breastfeeding either.

YOU MAY DEVELOP VARICOSE VEINS

Whilst these are not limited to pregnancy, it can certainly bring them on or exacerbate pre-existing ones. Varicose veins are swollen, enlarged veins that often have a bumpy and tortuous appearance. As well as being unsightly, they can cause itching and pain. They develop when the valves inside the veins become weakened or damaged and allow blood to flow backwards rather than to the heart, and the blood collects in the vein, giving them a swollen appearance. In pregnancy, there is extra strain on the veins due to the increased volume of blood, the pressure of the womb on the large vein (IVC), as well as the hormones causing the walls of the veins to become more lax, all making it more likely you will develop them. Whilst it is common to find varicose veins in your legs, in pregnancy, they can also develop in the pelvic area, sometimes affecting your vulva. Most women will find their varicose veins improve within a few months of the birth, but they may persist, and if they are causing you problems, there are possible treatment options available, including laser treatment, sclerotherapy (injecting a chemical into the vein to block it) and stripping (tying off and removing the vein).

YOUR BREASTS WILL CHANGE

During pregnancy, you will already have noticed changes to your breasts, with them becoming more tender or sensitive, larger, and changes in the colour and size of the nipples. After pregnancy, whether you breastfeed or not, your breasts probably won't look or feel the same as they used to, often changing in size and shape. I'll be honest with you, by day three postpartum, I looked like a porn star, with humongous breasts as my milk came in and hadn't quite regulated the required volume of milk needed. I also noticed the veins on my chest were more noticeable, and this is because of the increased blood volume. All household members were pretty chuffed with the new airbags; however, as time passed, the sag happened. They may now look like pancakes, but they served their purpose well, and they were always going to change as I went through different stages in my life. If, like me, you have two tennis balls swinging in a pair of socks, take solace in the fact that push-up bras exist. The important thing is to get used to how your 'new' breasts look and feel so that you can know your normal and identify when there are any changes.

YOUR LUSCIOUS PREGNANCY LOCKS WILL FALL

During pregnancy, the higher levels of oestrogen cause your hair to stay in the growing phase for longer than usual. This means that your hair tends to look thicker. In addition to this, in pregnancy you have an increased blood circulation, so your hair follicles may be delivered more nutrients and oxygen, making it healthier and grow better. So, by the time you give birth, your barnet is probably the bounciest and shiniest it's ever looked. Fast-forward 3 months and you are looking at your shower plug, wondering how that much hair can fall out without you actually being bald. This is because, after birth, your hormone levels normalise again, leading to a shift in the hair growth cycle, and more hairs enter the telogen (resting) phase, leading to the loss of the hairs that were previously stuck in the growing phase. It can feel scary to see that much hair fall out, but this is normal and, most important, temporary, and can last 6 to 12 months.

PERIODS BABY'S HERE

This is a huge topic for me, as I spent the best of 3 months speaking to gynaecology colleagues and reading every study and research paper there was about the return of periods postnatally. I did this because it took exactly 2 years and 3 months (who's counting, eh?!) for mine to return, and with every month that went by I panicked, thinking 'is this still normal?!'.

WHEN WILL YOUR PERIODS RETURN?

The answer to the question of when your periods will return depends largely on whether you breastfeed or not. For non-breastfeeding women, the first period can come as early as 6–8 weeks after delivery (sooner in some cases), though it can still take several months for them to return to a normal and regular cycle.

For those that breastfeed, the timing for your periods to resume varies hugely. The degree by which breastfeeding suppresses ovulation, and therefore your period, can depend on factors including the frequency and duration of breastfeeding and the baby's age. When exclusively breastfeeding (that is, no formula), including overnight, the likelihood of return of ovulation in the first 6 months is low (hence breastfeeding being an effective form of contraception). Still, once you start introducing solids or other fluids into your baby's diet at the 6-month mark, the breastfeeding frequency tends to become less, and therefore the chance of ovulation and a return of your period increases.

If you need more precise numbers, like me, the literature varies significantly. The largest study I found (834 patients) suggested the following timeframes, though it was published in 1951, so the numbers may not be as accurate for the woman of today, and it doesn't seem to reflect what we know now about lactational amenorrhoea for the first 6 months[145].

Return of period	Exclusively breastfeeding	Partly breastfeeding	Non-breastfeeding
Within 6 weeks postpartum		35.5%	47.3%
6–12 weeks postpartum	25.7%	51.3%	45.4%
12–18 weeks	20%		
18–24 weeks	14.3%		

This study also found that the earlier the return of your period, the more irregular it was.

Another much smaller study (of only 10 bottle-feeding and 27 breastfeeding mothers), also published decades ago, in 1982, found that on average periods returned at 8+/-1 weeks in bottle feeders and 32 +/-5 weeks in breastfeeders[146].

The inconsistency and variability in the statistics, and the lack of more recent research, does not help to prepare us for the expected return of our periods, but the studies do all agree that a return of periods is significantly sooner in bottle-feeding mothers.

However, as explained, mine returned significantly later, likely due to the ongoing frequency of night feeds (and my geriatric age, which I prefer to gloss over), so do not be disheartened if you do not fall neatly into the above statistics, but discuss it with your doctor if you have concerns.

WHAT WILL YOUR PERIODS BE LIKE?

They may feel different to how they were before. As my periods returned so much later than my other antenatal group mums, I was privy to all their experiences. Although I desperately wanted the return of my periods, I was also apprehensive about the deluge of blood and pain they described. But when they finally came, they were wonderful! I always had pain in the first 2 to 3 days, which wore me down, but on their recommencement, I felt absolutely nothing! If it weren't for the blood itself, I would have no indication that I was on my period. Your periods may differ in the following ways:

Flow – it may be heavier or lighter than before, though more commonly the first bleed tends to be heavier and longer.

Pain – you may develop more painful periods or, like me, they may become less painful. They tend to become more painful due to the increase in prostaglandins. This is a hormone released during your period and after childbirth that causes the womb to contract and cramp. In the postpartum period, the prostaglandin levels in the womb are higher than usual, which can cause more intense cramping. One theory as to why it may be less painful for some is that, somehow, during childbirth, some of the prostaglandin receptors in the womb are eliminated, resulting in fewer cramps.

Regularity – the significant hormonal changes that you go through postnatally can impact the regularity of your menstrual cycle and it may take several months before they become more regular and predictable.

RETURNING TO EXERCISE   BABY'S HERE

During pregnancy, I didn't stop exercising and, if anything, being in the pandemic and doing remote clinics from home and then being on maternity leave meant that I was exercising more than I ever had before. I remember thinking, whilst rubbing my baby bump and lunging in my garden, about how I wanted to get back to exercise as soon as possible after the birth. I enthusiastically googled 'Local mum and baby exercise classes' and expected to utilise the baby's 3kg weight for a more impactful squat. Enter Harris, and priorities change.

I was in such a bubble of new motherhood that I didn't even leave the house for the first 5 days after birth. Ordinarily, that would be my living hell, but it went in a flash. Eventually, I showered and realised I probably should let my new child see something of the world, so I took a short walk around our local green (I live in London, so its entire perimeter is only 400 metres). It felt good, but I didn't have a sudden physical activity awakening, and I was happy to return to the house and potter about after. For some, even a short walk may feel too much, and that is entirely ok; take it at your own pace.

Regular exercise after birth can aid physical recovery, increase much-needed energy levels, improve mood, help manage weight (though in the immediate postnatal period this is not necessarily a priority) and enhance your general wellbeing. I recommend beginning with gentle exercises and gradually increasing the intensity and duration.

Light exercises like walking, gentle movements, stretching, diaphragmatic breathing and pelvic floor exercising can be started as soon as you feel ready to, and these can help to rebuild your core strength, tone muscles and improve your cardiovascular fitness. However, there is no medal to be achieved by pushing your body further than feels comfortable, and it can do more harm than good. Be mindful of any pain or discomfort, and take breaks if you are feeling fatigued. Listen to your body, and if it doesn't feel right, stop or modify the exercise.

It is usually advised that you wait until your 6–8-week postnatal check before you begin any high-impact sports. An indication that you might be pushing it too hard too soon is that your lochia (the postnatal bleeding) can become heavier or change colour after activity, so pare back if this is the case. Whilst swimming is not considered high impact, it might be advisable to wait until your lochia has stopped or become less heavy and ensure that any wounds (C-section or episiotomy/tears) are well healed before your first tentative hop into the pool.

It is also important to remember that the hormone relaxin is still working its magic on your ligaments, so they will be looser and more lax for up to 5 months postnatally. This will be even longer in breast-feeding mothers, who will continue to produce relaxin whilst they breastfeed. You may start acing your yoga classes, getting into your downward dog position with far more ease, but it can also increase your risk of injuries.

If breastfeeding, you might find that higher-impact exercising can be uncomfortable with milk-laden boobs, so consider giving your baby a feed or pumping before you exercise to minimise the discomfort. Exercise alone won't negatively impact breast milk supply, however, it can alter the content slightly, though this is temporary and it will revert back to normal within a few hours. Dehydration, however, can affect breast milk supply, so ensuring adequate fluid and nutritional intake to balance the output of training is important as an imbalance can result in decreased milk production. In addition, nursing before exercise avoids the possible issue of increased milk acidity secondary to any lactic acid build-up. Investing in a supportive nursing sports bra is also much needed.

In the end, I didn't join any formal exercise classes, I simply walked for hours carrying Harris in a sling (my little koala only slept when attached to me), trying to keep the walks as brisk as possible, and when I had moments of peace at home, I would do some yoga or follow online postnatal exercise videos. This is all I felt my body needed for the first 6 months. At that 6+-month mark, something changed, and I felt ready for more, so I started using a running buggy, and Harris would come with me for little runs in the park. It took me an entire year before I went back to the HIIT classes that I was doing pre-pregnancy, and I look back, and I don't regret a moment of taking it slow. I have a pelvic floor that functions, a lower back that doesn't ache, and no injuries to be mindful of.

MANAGING UNSOLICITED ADVICE BABY'S HERE

You will get an endless stream of unsolicited advice from your family, neighbours, friends and random people who pester you on the street. It is not that this only happens in the newborn phase. Indeed, I'm not sure it ever stops, but you become much better at handling it and your confidence as a parent grows as time moves on. It is often very well-intentioned, but it can feel so overwhelming and even conflicting, adding to what is already a confusing and vulnerable time in your life. You are, of course, the expert on your child; no one knows them better, and you should always make decisions based on your own values, needs and beliefs, but it is rarely worth creating a drama with a well-meaning relative or friend over it. These are skills I have *tried* to master over the years in managing unsolicited advice:

Accept the emotions – it is entirely normal to feel annoyed when you receive unsolicited advice. You don't need to suppress those feelings, and by acknowledging them you are more likely to be able to manage and cope with them.

Trust your instincts – as a new parent, it can be so easy to default to the 'well, they probably know better' stance, but you have a unique insight into your baby, so rely on your instincts as the primary caregiver who knows your baby best.

Give them a chance – it can be so easy to jump on the defensive when you feel you are being criticised, but try to listen as they may be offering valuable advice. I suggest just filtering the advice that resonates with you and aligns with your own parenting philosophies and ignoring those that don't.

Practise a response – if you disagree with advice being given to you, respond assertively and confidently, thanking them for their input. You can say that you are following the guidance of your healthcare provider or have chosen a different approach that works for your family, or you can offer a non-committal response like 'interesting', remembering that you don't owe anyone an explanation for your choices.

Educate yourself – by seeking reliable sources like your healthcare provider or reputable parenting books and websites, you can be more confident and validated in your responses to those offering their differing advice. You may even be able to help educate the 'teacher'.

Set boundaries – you can try to be honest and let them know that while you appreciate their concern and support, you would prefer to figure things out independently, only being offered advice if you ask for it.

Master redirection – you can try to steer clear of a topic all you like, but sometimes you can still find yourself in a situation where unsolicited advice becomes overwhelming. In this case, redirect the conversation, perhaps towards positive aspects of parenting or heartwarming stories about your baby's milestones. If all else fails, stand up and offer to get coffee.

Find a support network – surround yourself with like-minded friends who share your values and have had similar experiences, or supportive individuals who respect your decisions and provide encouragement without imposing their views.

You will note the '*tried*' in the paragraph above, I was certainly not perfect, and I will end this section with a time that I am less than proud of how I handled a situation of unsolicited advice. Harris was 4 or 5 months old and would only be happy when attached to me. I didn't mind this most of the time, to be honest; I was often at my happiest, too, when I knew he was safe, warm and cosy, wrapped in a sling on my chest. However, after our weekly swimming lessons, I needed him to be in the pram, as he was often still a little wet and cold, and he would need to be wrapped up warm, and he wouldn't really fit bundled in a sling with layers on, especially with my wet hair dripping on him. I knew the pattern. Every Friday morning, after our swimming lesson, I would feed him, and he would be placed in the pram, where he would cry and whimper for the best part of the 15-minute walk it would take to get back home. I felt guilty, but I knew it was a short journey, that he always survived it, that it was for his own good, and I also knew that he would often fall asleep by the end of it. It would be a treat for me to have him sleep in the pram so I could get a few tasks done, and by the end of his sleep he would awake the happy chappy that he otherwise always was. One particular Friday, as I was making my walk back home, he was crying, and I was trying my best, as always, to soothe him, sing, stroke him and offer him a distraction, and I was tapped on the shoulder by a 50-something-year-old. I turned around to a scowling face who scolded, 'Why are you just letting your baby cry? There is something wrong with him!' At this point, I should have politely just said, 'Thank you for your concern, please don't worry, he is ok', and walked away. But rage filled every crevice of my body. My heart rate shot up, my face flushed and I spat the words, 'Excuse me? How dare you?' This of course did not de-escalate the situation, which together with the stillness of the pram, made Harris cry with even more ferocity and added further dramatics to the situation. She then told me that by not caring about him crying

I was making my child ill, that I should take him to a doctor, that I am an unfit mother, etc., etc. You get the drift. After a few more venomous back and forths, I regrettably told her to F-off, which she thankfully did. I picked Harris up out of his pram, awkwardly carrying him and pushing the pram the rest of the way back, and then, on arriving home, I sat with him on the sofa and cried waterfalls for a solid hour. I remember this event more than most of the lovely things that happened to our family that year, and I wish I had just let it go and not risen to it. Her words still haunt me. Unfit mother.

FIND YOUR CREW BABY'S HERE

I always read on various parenting sites: 'It takes a village to raise a child.' It's a quote that Hillary Clinton brought to the masses, but it originates as an African proverb. I've read it so many times it has almost lost its meaning, and I often wonder, when I'm in the depths of parenting hell, where is my village!? But in our modern world, the 'village' is more of an ecosystem of individuals, including the parents, wider family, teachers, healthcare professionals and friends, that interplay to keep our children happy and healthy.

We don't all have family we can rely on; our friends have their own lives to attend to and, as a GP, I know only too well how difficult it can be to get an appointment with a healthcare professional, let alone one just to have a rant and a moan about how many muslins you have to wash in a 24-hour period. As such, for the majority, your best bet in setting up your tribe is to find others at a similar place in their journey of parenthood. Despite my job and flaunting myself about on TV, I am such an introvert. The thought of having to put myself out there to awkwardly make new friends in my thirties was terrifying, but the saving grace is that everyone is in the same position, and everyone is desperate to make new mum friends to offload and relate to.

Antenatal classes are a good place to start, but if you didn't do antenatal classes (or you had a dud class with no one you got on with), there are plenty of other places to meet newbies like yourself in the postnatal world too. The first place to look is at postnatal classes. These may take the shape of sensory classes, music classes, swimming classes or rhyme time, to name a few. Make no mistake; these classes are for you. Your newborn, which can hardly see past its own fist, and whose only real desire is to be close to you and a milk source, couldn't care less about the man parading around with a monkey puppet on his hand and a disingenuous smile on his face, blaring out songs about swinging from trees. You, on the other hand, need this man, or, more precisely, the gravitational pull he has towards mums with babes. These postnatal classes are a networking hive, where parents almost always get there early to bond in the queue and then stay behind to swap numbers and pray someone will invite you for a coffee. If you attend regularly enough, some perfect mother with far greater organisational skills than you will ever have will create a WhatsApp group that will become your lifeline for all questions, reassurance and general moaning about your partner or baby. Remember that many of these classes can be done for free at children's centres or for a small donation at play-groups, so you do not need to pay through the nose to buy these friendships.

If classes aren't your thing, try public spaces. I know that sounds bizarre and, truthfully, you do feel a little like a weird mum predator, but I have met and exchanged numbers with so many mums I met loitering around parks, cafes and on the tube. Conversations nearly always begin with the customary 'oh cute, how old is your little one?' and hey presto the magic words are spoken and you have a new friend.

Finally, go online. There are numerous support groups out there, so tap into some of those in your local area. You will also be surprised at what a tight knit community the Instamums are, and there are plenty of Facebook groups dedicated to parenting, so put yourself out there and ask for some local recommendations. Even if, like me, you live in a city like London, and ordinarily find any stranger that talks to you majorly creepy, you will find that suddenly people, including yourself, are so much more friendly when they are on maternity leave and lonely. Embrace it and find your crew.

I also want to give a shout out to all those mums who had to go back to work early, or adoptive parents who don't get the full maternity leave, and therefore may feel like they have missed out on this opportunity to make friends. Don't underestimate the power of the nursery run. Whilst you wait at the nursery gate for the staff to open the Fort Knox-style security system, you will be surrounded by other parents who are also frantically trying to juggle their work and childcare. They will understand your plight, so use those precious moments to form the 'working mum clique'.

PRACTISING SELF-CARE BABY'S HERE

Realistically, in the early months, you won't be booking facials and massages, or a stylish brunch, wearing high heels. You will have unwashed hair, three-day-old pyjamas with posset on them, and you will be grateful if you can sit on the loo without an interruption. Therefore, let us change the pre-pregnancy narrative of self-care to more achievable post-pregnancy goals.

Schedule 'you' time – obviously, your newborn is your priority, but your ability to care for them in the compassionate way that you undoubtedly want to will hinge on your own sanity. So, take time out that is only yours. This can be as little as 5 minutes, if that is all that can be afforded, but know that every 6pm, or whatever time works for your family, you will have this time to do whatever it is you want, even if it is just to scroll through Instagram mindlessly, put on a face cream, play the piano or brush a serum through your hair. If anyone dares to disturb you, scream uncontrollably at them 'this is protected mummy time!' and with any luck the outburst will buy you a few more minutes.

Ask for help – not even the most in-control mothers out there can do it alone. Asking for help can come in the form of prompting a friend to empty the washing machine, a family member to watch over your baby whilst you shower, a partner to let you catch up on sleep, or a neighbour to cook a meal. It is not a sign of failure to ask for help, you are expected at this stage to need help. If you are struggling with processing any emotions, reach out for emotional help from friends, a therapist or a support group. Seeking professional help isn't indulgent, it's a vital part of self-care.

Connect – when you have a baby, everyone comes out of the woodwork to congratulate you. Some of these people will support and uplift you, others will drain you. Your energy levels at this point are critical, so allow yourself the confidence to surround yourself with those who bring positivity and politely decline connecting with those that bring you down.

Sleep – I hate that I am writing this down, because every time I read it when I had a newborn, I wanted to hurl the screen/book at the wall, but you should try to 'sleep when they sleep'. I personally found this impossible for several reasons. Firstly, because my child only wanted to contact nap, and I would always be in the most uncomfortable positions wedged between pillows and sofas, which were entirely unsafe places to co-sleep. Secondly, because if I ever did manage to get him to sleep in a cot, I would have a reel of tasks I needed to do whilst he was asleep playing over and over in my head so that sleep would not come no matter how tired I was. Lastly, because I was an obsessed mother who missed her child when he slept, even if I had the intention to sleep I would end up looking through photos of him on my phone and crying over how much he has changed in seven days. Having said all of this, I would still recommend trying to prioritise your own sleep. It is a fundamental aspect of self-care, and it is crucial for your overall wellbeing and ability to function. If sleeping when they sleep is impossible, try to schedule it in other ways. I used to pass Harris over to Rupert at 5.30/6am every morning for an hour and a half before he had to start work, and I would sleep the deepest, most-needed sleep of my life. I truly believe those one and a half hours were the only things that kept me alive in those first few months.

Self-compassion – recognise that it is entirely normal to experience a wide range of emotions after having a baby, whether you're overwhelmed, anxious, exhausted, frustrated or sad. Acknowledge these feelings, and understand it is ok to have ups and downs without judgement. You're doing the best you can; you will make mistakes, but treat yourself with the kindness and understanding that you would your friend or loved one. By practising self-compassion and acting in a nurturing and supportive way with yourself, you can positively impact your own wellbeing and your ability to care for your baby.

Eat well – establishing healthy eating habits in the postpartum period will help
with your recovery, energy levels and your general wellbeing. I certainly relied
heavily on pre-prepared frozen meals initially, so, where possible, batch-cook
some nutrient-dense foods so that you have healthy choices available when
time is short. To maintain steady energy levels throughout the day you may
also want to consider smaller, more frequent meals and snacks – make sure
these include a mix of proteins, healthy fats and fibre (nuts are always my
go-to snack). Don't forget to drink plenty of water to keep hydrated,
especially if you are breastfeeding.

Whatever form self-care takes, just remember to be patient as you
adjust to this transition. Focus on nourishing your body and mind and
resting when needed, but allow yourself some flexibility and grace.

POSTNATAL, BABY AND YOU: A TIRED MAMMA'S SUMMARY

APGAR score: the quick assessment of a newborn's health known as the APGAR
score, which evaluates appearance, pulse, grimace, activity and respiration.
This score helps determine the baby's overall wellbeing and potential need for
special care.

Skin-to-skin contact: the benefits of skin-to-skin contact between mother and
baby (and father and baby) include its positive impact on breastfeeding
initiation, temperature regulation, stress reduction and bonding.

Vitamin K: a vitamin K injection is offered to prevent bleeding disorders in
newborns, there is also an option for oral doses.

Cord clamping/cutting: the process of clamping and then cutting the umbilical
cord after your baby is born. There are benefits to delayed cord clamping,
particularly in transferring iron to the newborn and enhancing overall health.

Perineal tears and episiotomy: tips for managing pain, discomfort and healing
from perineal tears and episiotomies can include pain relief, ice packs,
'padsicles', the use of a peri-bottle, good hygiene and infection prevention.

Newborn health checks: the Newborn and Infant Physical Examination (NIPE) screening programme aims to identify congenital abnormalities of the eyes, heart, hips and testes within 72 hours of birth. The NIPE screening is repeated at 6–8 weeks after birth by the GP to further detect congenital abnormalities.

Caesarean recovery: the average stay in hospital after a Caesarean section is 2–4 days. The recovery process usually takes around 6 weeks.

Blood spot test (heel prick test): a blood test taken from your baby's heel that screens for rare but serious conditions in newborns.

Cord care: midwives check the baby's umbilical cord for signs of health, drying and infection during postnatal visits. Parents are advised to keep the cord clean and dry until it naturally falls off, 1 to 3 weeks after birth.

Jaundice: yellow discoloration of the skin and eyes, common in newborns due to bilirubin (a chemical made from the breakdown of red blood cells) buildup. It is usually harmless, but some babies need phototherapy to reduce its levels.

6–8-week postnatal check: postnatal checkup with a GP to monitor the mother's recovery after childbirth, covering both physical and mental health concerns.

Postnatal depression and baby blues: both baby blues and postnatal depression can affect mood after the birth of your baby, but they are different. Whilst baby blues is transient, postnatal depression persists and may need the support of groups, mindfulness techniques, therapy and medication.

Sex and contraception: your libido can be affected for a number of reasons postnatally, and this is normal. Go at your own speed and don't feel pressured to have sex. There are different contraceptive options available, including hormonal methods, intrauterine contraception, barrier methods and sterilisation.

PHYSICAL BODY CHANGES

Body appearance: it's normal for a woman's body to still look pregnant after childbirth, due to factors like womb shrinking, retained fluid and abdominal muscle recovery.

Hip and rib cage changes: a woman's hips and rib cage may be wider after pregnancy, due to hormonal changes and increased space needed for the growing womb. While these changes usually revert to normal, it may vary among individuals.

Caesarean section healing: abdominal strength recovery takes time, progress gradually with physical activities to avoid injury.

Skin changes: including linea nigra (dark vertical line on the abdomen), increased pigmentation and stretch marks.

Diastasis recti: the separation of abdominal muscles during pregnancy.

Breast changes: changes in size, shape and skin appearance occur during pregnancy and postpartum. Embrace these changes and find ways to adapt, such as using supportive bras.

Hair loss: occurs after pregnancy due to hormonal shifts, this is temporary and normal.

Return of menstruation: there is variation in when and how periods may return after childbirth, with factors like breastfeeding and individual variations affecting this. You may notice changes in flow, pain and regularity.

Returning to exercise: start gentle exercises after birth and gradually increase intensity. Factors affecting exercise include hormone levels, ligament laxity and breastfeeding considerations.

CHAPTER 7

FEEDING YOUR BABY

I think it is fair to say that decisions around feeding our babies are rarely straightforward. This is such an emotive topic. Breastfeeding gave me immense joy for the most part, but for so many it is connected with sadness, anger, guilt or fear. It's a little terrifying to navigate a chapter that discusses something with such broad emotions associated with it, yet it needs to be talked about. Not enough mothers talk about it.

Hammering into mums-to-be or new mums all the benefits of breastfeeding may convert a number of women who weren't sure if they wanted to breastfeed, or continue to breastfeed, but there will be many reading this who will find hearing about this meaningless at best and triggering at worst. That's because those that wanted to breastfeed their babies but couldn't, for whatever reason, may feel that their preferred method of feeding was in effect stolen from them, often because they were unsupported to overcome the reasons behind it. They may also feel guilt that their babies are missing out on these benefits. So it is ok to skip to the bottle and formula feeding section at the end of this chapter if you are struggling with breastfeeding; self-preservation is important.

Whether you intend to breastfeed, are struggling with breastfeeding now, already know that you don't want to breastfeed, or aren't sure of your intentions, it is always worth arming yourself with knowledge. Whether reading my book or seeking it from other reputable resources, do your homework; breastfeeding is a minefield.

THE PHYSIOLOGY OF BREASTFEEDING
BE PREPARED

Whilst I'm sure many of you are not here for an anatomy or science lesson, I hope that by demystifying the process and physiology of breastfeeding, the knowledge and understanding will empower you with confidence in this amazing and natural process.

The breasts begin to develop during puberty, but the entire ductal system needed for breastfeeding does not mature until pregnancy, when hormonal changes trigger it. The oestrogen promotes the development of milk ducts (a network of thin tubes) which are required for the storage and delivery of milk, and progesterone promotes the development of the lobules and alveoli (hollow sacs), which are responsible for milk production. When breastfeeding, the ducts carry the milk from the alveoli towards the areola (the dark area of skin in the middle of your breasts), where the ducts all join together into larger ducts that end at the nipple.

In the second half of pregnancy the hormone prolactin increases and triggers off colostrum production. However, the placenta is producing high levels of progesterone, which inhibits significant lactation, so only small amounts of colostrum can be expressed at this point. This is known as Stage I Lactogenesis. Once the placenta is delivered after birth, there is a sudden drop in progesterone and the uninhibited high prolactin triggers copious lactation (Stage II Lactogenesis).

When the newborn then starts to suckle or you start pumping, there is a surge in the hormone oxytocin, which causes a milk ejection reflex, also known as a 'let down', where the milk travels from the alveoli into the milk ducts, allowing the baby to drink. On emptying the alveoli, prolactin then activates the milk-producing cells (the lactocytes) in the alveoli, triggering off even more milk production. This therefore means that the more frequent the nipple stimulation and let down, the more milk is produced. It is a wonderful example of positive feedback, ensuring that the milk we make equals the baby's requirement. Where the milk is not removed, the feedback system inhibits the effect of prolactin, and milk production stops. This ongoing milk supply, emptying and feedback control is Stage III Lactogenesis.

BREAST MILK COMPOSITION BE PREPARED

Breast milk contains everything a baby needs up until 6 months of life, including water, fat, carbohydrates, proteins, vitamins and minerals. It also contains immune components to help them fight infections and other factors to aid digestion and the absorption of nutrients.

COLOSTRUM

Colostrum secreted in the first 2–3 days contains higher concentrations of the immune components, protein, minerals and vitamins (A, E, K) than later milk. Colostrum helps to coat and seal the gut lining, which is more leaky (permeable) when babies are born, and it acts like a laxative in allowing the passage of the meconium more easily. You will only produce small amounts (40–50ml in 24 hours), but it isn't known as liquid gold for nothing – it might be tiny, but it is mighty, and it is all your baby needs.

TRANSITIONAL MILK

Once the milk is said to have 'come in' 2–4 days after delivery, milk is produced in larger amounts and your breasts will feel bigger and fuller. At this point, your baby will be drinking between 300 and 400ml every 24 hours, and that will go up to 500–800ml by day five. By days 5–14, the milk is called transitional and becomes more calorific, being higher in fat and lactose[147].

MATURE MILK

After 2 weeks it is called mature milk, and the nutritional content and levels of ingredients in mature milk generally remain fairly consistent. But the composition of your breast milk is still dynamic and can change from day to day and feed to feed. It can be influenced by your diet, hydration, the baby's nursing patterns and the time of day. Interestingly, the composition of the milk can also depend on the baby's maturity. The breast milk of mothers to premature babies typically contains higher protein concentrations, proportional to the degree of prematurity.

FOREMILK AND HINDMILK

This used to be a thing. Foremilk and hindmilk were terms used to describe the different compositions in milk during a feed. Foremilk refers to the milk produced at the beginning of the feed that tends to be more watery, lower in fat, but high in lactose, proteins, vitamins and minerals. Whereas hindmilk refers to the milk produced towards the end of the feed, which is thicker and has a higher fat content.

However, we have moved away from these terms, mainly because they oversimplify the process. It implies that there are two distinct and separate compositions but it is more complex than that, and we now know that it varies gradually throughout the feed. Foremilk and hindmilk are not separate types of milk produced by different glands; they are different stages of the same milk. The emphasis on foremilk and hindmilk often led to anxiety in mothers about whether they were getting the right balance of the two types. Recent research, though, suggests that if you allow your baby to feed responsively on demand and for as long as they need to over 24 hours, your baby will consume fairly consistent amounts of fat each day[148]. The growth of your baby will ultimately be determined by overall calories consumed, rather than the specific concentration of fat, so focusing too much on the fat itself rather than overall volume of milk consumed is counterproductive.

THE BENEFITS OF BREASTFEEDING   BE PREPARED

The benefits of breastfeeding extend beyond just nutrition and immune protection, it also provides an emotional connection, as well as longer-term health benefits to both the mother and child.

BENEFITS TO YOUR BABY

Nutrition – breast milk offers the optimal balance of proteins, carbohydrates, fats, vitamins and minerals, which adapts to the baby's changing nutritional needs as they grow. The baby's immature digestive system easily digests the proteins in breast milk, and it contains enzymes to further aid digestion and nutrient absorption. This means breast fed babies are less likely to suffer with digestive issues like constipation and diarrhoea.

Immune support – breast milk contains a number of immune components, including antibodies, white blood cells, enzymes and other immune factors. These help protect the baby from infections and diseases, which is especially important in the early months when their immune system is still so immature. This may reduce the risk of developing respiratory, gastrointestinal, ear and urinary tract infections, to name a few. It also contains prebiotics to nourish the beneficial gut bacteria and contribute to a healthy gut microbiome, which in turn helps the development of their own defences.

Reduced risk of chronic disease – evidence suggests that breastfed babies have a reduced risk of developing chronic diseases like obesity, type 2 diabetes, asthma and cardiovascular disease in adulthood[149].

Cognitive development – breastfeeding has been linked to higher IQ scores and improved cognitive development in children[150].

Regulation – breastfeeding can have a calming effect on the baby due to the close contact, the rhythmic suckling and the calming effects of the hormones within breast milk. This can help regulate their emotions and give them a sense of security.

BENEFITS TO YOU

Convenience – it's always there whenever you need it. It's available, at the right temperature, does not involve sterilising and, of course, it is free.

Emotional connection – there is a sense of closeness that develops when you breastfeed. This can occur because of the physicality of the skin-to-skin contact and the frequent eye contact. But there is also an element of mutual understanding. You learn to understand your baby's cues and needs to satisfy hunger and comfort, which strengthens your emotional bond and fosters trust. Hormones, of course, also play their part, as the oxytocin released during breastfeeding helps to foster feelings of love, and prolactin can contribute to the feelings of protectiveness, nurturing instincts and attachment towards the baby. It is imperative to note, though, that breastfeeding is not the only way to establish a strong emotional connection with a baby, and cuddling, playing, soothing and simple responsive caregiving can also harbour that bond.

Recovery – the oxytocin released during breastfeeding causes the womb to contract after birth, reducing the risk of postpartum bleeding, therefore helping the mother's recovery.

Reduced risk of chronic disease – breastfeeding has been shown to reduce the risk of cardiovascular disease, type 2 diabetes, breast cancer, ovarian cancer, womb cancer, osteoporosis and obesity. It also reduces the risk of postpartum depression[151, 152, 153].

Contraception – as discussed previously (see section on contraception), you can use exclusive breastfeeding as a form of contraception in the first 6 months after birth. It may also mean your periods stay away longer, which is a bonus if you normally have painful or heavy periods.

THE DOWNSIDES OF BREASTFEEDING
BE PREPARED

I wouldn't be being honest or balanced if I didn't talk about the negatives of breastfeeding. It's amazing in so many respects, but I found the sole responsibility of breastfeeding quite overwhelming at times. In the first few months it is full on, and when they are cluster feeding, it can be a huge drain on your energy and time. As the baby's sole source of nutrition, breastfeeding anchors you to your baby. This is probably what you naturally want anyway in those initial months, but as time progresses and you may feel the need for a little more autonomy and independence it can be more challenging.

There are, of course, ways to involve others through pumping, but often I felt it was just easier to breastfeed than spend time pumping, sterilising, defrosting and reheating. Whilst many women love pumping and the freedom it offers, I just felt like a dairy cow. I hated the loud, rhythmic noise that the electric pump made, the way you could see your nipple being sucked in and out through the see-through plastic attachments, the nakedness and vulnerability I felt when I had them on, and that I could see how much came out and inevitably felt a pang of anxiety when I wasn't sure there would be enough. I also really struggled to find a sanitary place to pump when I wasn't at home, and sitting in public loos pumping genuinely saddened me and made me want to run back to my baby and clean home.

I remember being on a media job and I had to spend the night away from my son for the first time when he was 5 months old. I specifically told them beforehand that I would need somewhere to pump between filming and was reassured this wouldn't be an issue. Cue the day and I was sitting in a freezing unisex warehouse toilet with my jumpsuit around my ankles. There were no electricity points so the electric pump wouldn't work, and I was hand expressing and holding back the tears lest I ruin the TV makeup! I'm certain that there would have been ways around all of these obstacles, and I am such an advocate of trying to address challenges in breastfeeding with support, guidance and education, but it's important to recognise that breastfeeding isn't always the breeze it's made out to be.

Breastfeeding in public should not have to be here in my list of cons of breastfeeding, and yet in 2023 it is. In the first few months, I felt self-conscious and I used a breastfeeding cover, after that I felt more confident and did away with it. Mostly, people would ignore me, or I would get a brief smile or approving nod of the head, though occasionally I would hear a tut or see a disapproving head shake, often from the older population, but the ease of it all superseded any rare negative judgements.

However, as Harris got older, there was certainly a change in atmosphere. Extended breastfeeding was not accepted as readily as the feeding of an infant, and I felt increasingly uncomfortable, so I eventually decided only to feed Harris in the privacy of homes. As a confident woman, I'm almost ashamed to admit to the fact that I allowed other people's judgements of me to change my natural maternal behaviour. I can only imagine how a woman who perhaps feels less confident may curtail their breastfeeding journey early to avoid social stigma and judgement.

As part of the issue with autonomy, the restrictions that breastfeeding can put on your diet and lifestyle can also be a barrier. You often find yourself limiting alcohol and caffeine, and avoiding more than two portions of oily fish. Similar to pregnancy, you are still restricted with many medications, skincare products and aesthetic treatments. Though be aware that alternatives can be found to many of these perceived restrictions.

I will discuss pain further in the troubleshooting section (page 204), but not everyone has an easy breastfeeding journey, and it can be peppered with sore nipples, engorgement and mastitis, which can all make breastfeeding uncomfortable. Tongue tie can also affect your breastfeeding journey, which is not always picked up early during the newborn examinations. It can sometimes only become obvious once there is an issue with feeding. Most of these issues have solutions and ways to reduce the risk of developing them, but when you are in the midst of it all, and it feels like razor blades on your nipples every time your baby drinks, it can be so emotionally and physically draining.

Lastly, milk supply can be a challenge. Producing too little milk can lead to anxiety about your baby's nutrition. Conversely, producing too much can lead to issues with engorgement and difficulty for your baby to feed. With support and intervention we can often regulate the supply, but the journey to get to that point can be incredibly frustrating.

Breastfeeding mantras

There is no doubt that breastfeeding is beneficial, however, individual circumstances and preferences vary, and considering a mother's and baby's health, lifestyle and overall wellbeing is equally important. This is why the mantra 'breast is best' is highly outdated.

Although it had been used, probably quite innocently, to encourage women to breastfeed as the preferred method of feeding, it can inadvertently induce the feeling of guilt, inadequacy and judgement for not breastfeeding. It is a phrase that may overlook the complex reasons why some mothers are unable to or choose not to breastfeed.

Then the more inclusive phrase 'fed is best' was born, in the hope that mothers understood that, as a population, we recognised and respected that families come in different forms and have such varying feeding experiences. It focused on ensuring all babies received optimal nutrition and care, regardless of whether they are breast- or formula-fed. Again, the intention was good, but it did not necessarily include the group of women who desperately wanted to breastfeed, who felt saddened and angry at their unsuccessful journey, and perhaps felt dismissed by everyone who would shrug them off with the phrase 'fed is best'.

Enter 'informed is best'. The emphasis here is on providing accurate, evidence-based information, resources and support for both breastfeeding and formula-feeding parents, allowing parents to make informed decisions about feeding their babies. This mantra aims to highlight the benefits of breastfeeding whilst respecting that it may not be possible or desired by everyone. It also encourages parents to educate themselves, speak to healthcare professionals and lactation consultants, and make informed decisions that take into consideration the wellbeing of both the baby and the parents.

HOW TO PREPARE FOR BREASTFEEDING
BE PREPARED

I had done no preparation in the lead up to breastfeeding aside from attending my Zoom antenatal class, in which I vaguely remember them telling me something about latching on a knitted breast (I'm sure they taught me more, but in my late-pregnant stage I was probably popping out the room for toilet breaks, biccies and tea, and zoning out!).

However, with my retrospective hat on, I do believe that you need to be mentally and physically prepared for breastfeeding.

Information is your ally – your antenatal class should cover positioning, latch, expressing and the common breastfeeding issues that arise, so take notes to refer back to when you are in a breastfeeding crisis. If you don't choose to attend antenatal classes, you can source information in books, support groups and reputable online resources. Your midwife and health visitor can also help answer any questions you have, so write them all down in preparation for your appointments (both antenatally and postnatally). If you have any breastfeeding friends, hang out with them and learn what 'normal' looks like. However, also note how varied breastfeeding patterns and behaviours can be, to reassure you that it might just take time before you and your baby become comfortable with your unique rhythm of breastfeeding.

Prepare all your supplies – before the baby arrives, make room for a dedicated boob drawer, stocking up on nursing bras, nursing pads, nipple cream, clothes and PJs that allow for easy access, and gel packs to ease any discomfort. You may also want to consider a nursing pillow to help you to get into a comfortable position, and if you plan to pump then have a pump and milk storage bags. I also had a 'just in case' stash of formula. I know some people don't recommend this defeatist attitude, but for me it was never defeatist, only practical in preparing for all eventualities so that I wasn't sending my husband out in a blind panic at 3am to a petrol station to buy some. You are also able to prepare for the 'just in case' eventualities in the first few days by ensuring you have harvested colostrum and it's ready and waiting to be defrosted.

Set up a breastfeeding station – you can be stuck in a certain position feeding your baby and then be nap-trapped for a while, so you may as well make the position the best one you will ever be in! I had one end of a comfy sofa, with a nursing pillow, a blanket and a reachable side table with the remote control, drinks and snacks, phone charger and lanolin nipple cream. Don't underestimate how hungry and thirsty you get when breastfeeding and stock that side table high with healthy goodies. I also signed up to Netflix for three months and binge-watched a lifetime of trashy TV.

Have the right vitamins – there is no specific diet you need to follow for breastfeeding, but, like everyone, you should try to eat a well-balanced and healthy diet. The only food to be mindful of is fish. Whilst it is healthy for you and your baby, during breastfeeding you should not have more than two portions of fish a week, due to low-level pollutants that can build up in the body. You should also limit shark, swordfish or marlin, as they are higher in mercury. One of the few vitamins we often can't get enough of purely from diet is vitamin D. It is primarily made from a reaction of the sun on our skin, and is needed to regulate the calcium and phosphate in our body, ensuring healthy bones. It has also been implicated in other functions, including our immune system. In the UK, it is advised that everyone, including pregnant and breastfeeding women, should consider taking 10mg of vitamin D daily. This is especially important in the months between October and March when we are less able to get enough vitamin D from sunlight. However, research indicates that pregnant and lactating women might need more vitamin D than adults who are not bearing children[154], and thus you may want to consider taking it throughout breastfeeding.

HOW TO ESTABLISH A STRONG BREASTFEEDING RELATIONSHIP   BABY'S HERE

A positive breastfeeding relationship from the start is necessary for a successful journey. This may just be the need for some practical tips or techniques, or it may take the form of more formal support systems.

GET OFF TO A POSITIVE START

Practise skin-to-skin contact immediately after birth to promote bonding and encourage breastfeeding initiation. Commence breastfeeding as soon after birth as possible, as there is evidence to suggest that if you start within an hour of delivery it has a positive impact on the duration of exclusive breastfeeding[155]. Not only this, but feeding within an hour has also been shown to protect against infection and reduce neonatal death due to sepsis, pneumonia, diarrhoea and hypothermia[156].

OPTIMISE THE LATCH

Your baby latching onto your breast to feed may seem like a simple task, but it requires a few steps and doesn't always come naturally to all mothers and babies. However, it is a skill that can be learned:

1. Find a comfortable position for you and your baby.
2. If you have large breasts it can be helpful to support your breast with one hand, forming a 'C' shape with your fingers.
3. Bring your baby close to your body with their body in a straight line, aligning their nose with your nipple.
4. Their chin should be touching your breast, allowing the head to tip back to help them to get a deep latch. Make sure your hand isn't touching the back of their head.
5. They will open their mouth in a wide gape, which will help them to get a deep latch. Guide them towards the breast as they do this.
6. Ensure your baby has the darker area around the nipple (areola) in their mouth, not just the nipple.
7. Your baby should have an asymmetrical latch with more of the areola visible above the nipple than below.
8. It should not be painful, so if you are experiencing discomfort, gently put a clean finger in the corner of your baby's mouth to break the suction, then try latching again.

FIND THE RIGHT POSITION

There are a number of different positions that you can adopt with your baby when breastfeeding, and it is about finding which one works best for you both. There are four main feeding positions:

Cross cradle hold – this is the most commonly used position. It involves your baby lying across your body and supporting your baby's back with your forearm, and their head and neck with your hand, leaving the head free to tilt back and latch. Your baby's body will be facing you and they will be aligned so that their ear, shoulder and hip are in a straight line at the level of your breast.

You can use a nursing pillow to help support their body if that is your preference. Once your baby is deeply latched and transferring milk you can switch arms to use a classic cradle hold.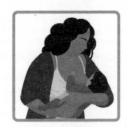

Rugby hold – this represents how you would hold a rugby ball, tucking your baby under your arm. You rest your arm on your side, on a pillow, with your baby's head supported by your hand and their legs extended behind you. This position is helpful if you have had a Caesarean section, when it may be uncomfortable to have your baby lie across your tummy. It can also be helpful if you have large breasts.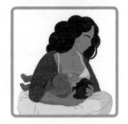

Side lying – this position became a firm favourite of mine for night feeds. It's also helpful if you have had a Caesarean and getting up can be sore. You lie on your side, with your baby lying on their side facing you, checking that they are aligned with their ear, shoulder and hip all in a straight line. Use your free arm to support your baby, then your other arm can go under your head or pillow (ensuring it is not too close to your baby's head).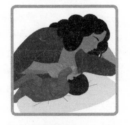

Laidback nursing – in this position you can recline with pillows supporting your back, neck and shoulders. Your baby lies on top of you, on their tummy, with your hands gently supporting them as they feed. This position promotes natural breastfeeding instincts and reflexes, which is why it is also known as 'biological nursing'.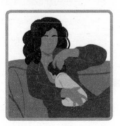

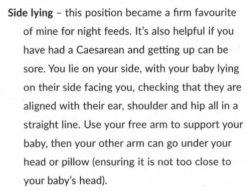

RECOGNISE HUNGER CUES

It is recommended that breastfed babies are fed responsively (on demand) and recognising hunger cues is a large part of that, though of course recognising hunger in bottle-fed babies is equally important. However, crying is often a late sign that they are hungry and babies exhibit more subtle cues before the meltdown to communicate their need for a feed. The cues can vary among newborns, so it may take time observing your baby before you identify their unique signals.

Early signs that your baby is hungry can include lip smacking, opening and closing their mouths, and sucking on their hands, fingers, toes, toys, or anything they can get their mouth on! Later signs include the rooting reflex, which occurs when a hungry baby instinctively turns their head towards anything that brushes against their cheek or the mouth, in the hope that they will find a nipple and start feeding. A way to test whether your child may be ready for a feed is to stroke their cheek and see if they turn their head and open their mouth. The rooting reflex usually disappears by 3 to 4 months old and it becomes voluntary. They may also start to become more active, fidgeting, fussing, squirming and pulling at your clothes, or rooting around on the chest of whoever is carrying them.

If these signs are missed, your baby may then cry or move their head frantically to communicate their hunger. Ideally, you want to identify the cues before they become too upset as they may not be able to feed effectively if they are not calm. It is also important to note that hunger is not the only reason a baby may want to breastfeed. Other factors like comfort, warmth and the need for oral stimulation can all be drivers for a baby to want to breastfeed.

BURP YOUR BABY

Whether your baby is breastfed or bottle-fed, when your baby feeds they tend to also swallow air, which can become trapped in their stomach, causing discomfort and excessive gas. Burping your baby after their feed helps them to expel that swallowed air, relieving the symptoms of discomfort and reducing the frequency of spitting up. It may also help to empty the stomach, making more room for milk and improving their feeding. There are a few different ways in which you can burp your baby:

Over your shoulder – hold your baby against your chest with their chin resting on your shoulder. Support their head with one hand and gently rub or pat their back in an upward motion with the other.

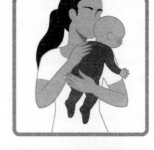

On your lap – whilst sitting down, sit your baby on your lap and lean them slightly forwards, with one hand against their chest and supporting their chin, and the other hand patting or rubbing their back.

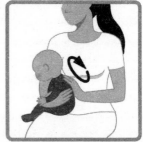

Lying across your lap – with your baby lying face down across your lap, support their chin with one hand and gently pat or rub their back with the other.

Wonky winding – essentially this is the left lateral position. In this position, you are holding your baby as you would against your chest for the over-the-shoulder position, but then you lean them to their left side. This technique is not often written about, but it is one that helped me a lot with Harris. Lyndsey Hookway, a paediatric nurse, coined this phrase when she was working long night shifts with sad and uncomfortable babies, and noticed that when she held the baby facing outwards on their left, they settled more. She wasn't some baby whisperer, rather she was using her knowledge of anatomy, which she explains:

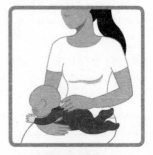

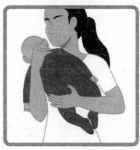

'The stomach is not circular, it is more the shape of a banana, and the highest point of the stomach is the fundus. As the fundus is the highest part of the stomach, gas can get trapped here. If the stomach is not overly full, or the baby is moving around independently, then often the gas can pass out fairly easily. However, babies spend a lot of their time on their backs, fairly immobile, feeding a lot, with a small stomach capacity, all of which can contribute to discomfort. If the stomach is full, holding them vertically to wind them doesn't often work because the trapped air in the fundus would need to travel down and then go up, and air doesn't do that. However, lying on the left means the highest point of the stomach is the oesophagus, not the fundus, so it's easier for the air to come out.'

It is worth pointing out that not all babies need burping. If a breast-fed baby is latched deeply, they may not swallow much air and therefore may not need to be winded. Certainly, see how your baby is after a feed, and try winding them if that settles them, but if they aren't unsettled or they are not bringing up any wind, then they may not need to be burped at all.

THE EVOLUTION OF THE BREASTFEEDING JOURNEY BABY'S HERE

This is an evolving journey, which will often look very different in the first few weeks to how it will look 6 months down the line when you are introducing solid foods, or years down, should you consider extended nursing. No matter the stage of breastfeeding, it is both an intimate and often demanding period of motherhood.

We have discussed the early days of colostrum, with short and frequent feeds to stimulate milk production. We have also discussed the milk 'coming in', establishing the milk supply in the transition to mature milk, and the necessity of overcoming any challenges like latching and positioning. But how does the rest of your journey unravel?

As your baby develops, their nutritional needs will change, but amazingly you don't have to do anything in those first six months. Your breast milk will remarkably adapt to meet these needs, providing the appropriate balance of nutrients. Whilst the lactose content, which is the primary carbohydrate in breast milk and which provides a steady source of energy for your baby, remains relatively consistent throughout lactation, other macronutrients change. The ratio of protein in breast milk shifts from whey to casein as lactation progresses. Whey is easier for a newborn to digest, this ratio moves towards casein, which provides a greater sense of fullness and supports growth as your baby develops. The fat content increases as your baby becomes more active and their energy requirements increase. Growth spurts may also prompt your baby to want more frequent feeds, which can require increased patience and ongoing responsivity from your side.

Breast milk not only adapts to your baby's age but also to their individual needs, including factors like their growth patterns, feeding behaviours and health. A remarkable feature of breast milk is to adapt immunologically in response to your baby's health. If, for example, a baby is exposed to a certain infection, the mother is able to detect the presence of the pathogens from the baby's saliva when it comes into contact with her during a breastfeed, and produce the appropriate antibodies in her breast milk to protect the baby.

At around 6 months of age you will introduce solid foods (see weaning, page 251) alongside breastfeeding. Initially, breast milk will remain the primary source of nutrition, but as your child starts to eat more, you may notice a reduction in the frequency and/or duration of feeds. Becoming more independent and mobile may also change the nature of your feeds, as your baby can start to become more distracted and make fewer demands for feeds.

When a parent chooses to stop breastfeeding varies significantly. The World Health Organisation recommends that all babies are breastfed exclusively for the first 6 months of life, and that from 6 months they should start eating solids alongside breastfeeding for 2 years and beyond.[157]

Extended breastfeeding is not particularly common, but a child's immune system is still developing until around age 5, so there are certainly benefits beyond nutrition and comfort. The last UK-wide infant feeding survey (in 2010) found that 81 per cent of women initiated breastfeeding, though this dropped to between 17–24 per cent by 6 weeks[158]. At 4 months it was 12 per cent and by 6 months only 1 per cent were still exclusively breastfeeding. Given the excellent initiation rates, I think the drop-off rates highlight the need to seek support, stay informed and practise self-care in the face of the challenges that breast-feeding might present along the way.

ALCOHOL AND BREASTFEEDING BE PREPARED

This topic comes up a lot in friendship groups, but honestly I am rarely asked about it in a GP setting. I suspect mothers are too worried about bringing up alcohol and breastfeeding with their GP lest they are judged. However, you have been essentially tee-total for 9 months, I think it's absolutely reasonable to want to know whether it is safe to drink again, and if so, how much. As with many 'taboo' topics, it is always better to talk about it openly and get an informed and educated answer than it is to just guess or blindly google.

The messaging from the RCOG broadly suggests a few drinks spread over the week is 'probably' safe. Their exact wording is: 'The safest option is to avoid alcohol during breastfeeding as alcohol can find its way into your breast milk. Regular drinking during breastfeeding may affect your baby's development. If you do choose to drink, it is safest not to drink more than 14 units per week and best to spread your drinks evenly during the week.'[159]

Let us begin with understanding the science behind it. The concentration of alcohol in breast milk is roughly equivalent to the concentration of alcohol in the mother's blood. To work out your Blood Alcohol Concentration (BAC), several factors are taken into account, including the amount of alcohol consumed, the mother's body weight (a higher body weight in general leads to a lower BAC for the same amount of alcohol consumed, as it is distributed more widely in a larger body), and the time elapsed since drinking. The liver metabolises and eliminates alcohol at a fairly consistent rate of roughly one unit (10ml or 8g of pure alcohol) an hour. Other more individual factors like the mother's metabolism, medication and general health can also contribute to the BAC. To give you an example, if you were a 65kg woman who had just drunk a glass (150ml) of 12 per cent wine, your BAC would be 0.033 per cent and it would take around 3 hours for it to reach 0 per cent. Ultimately, 0.033 per cent is a pretty miniscule amount of alcohol to enter your breast milk and into your baby, which is probably why the RCOG don't have a hard line about no alcohol, but as there is technically no 'safe' amount of alcohol we should be feeding our babies, the advice is murky. We must also be reminded that even though this percentage of alcohol is tiny, babies are also tiny, and newborns break down alcohol more slowly than adults, metabolising alcohol at 20–25 per cent the rate at which we can[160]. This means that the alcohol stays in their bodies for longer.

However, there are ways that you can limit your baby's exposure should you fancy a tipple:

- It can take up to 2–3 hours for a standard drink to be processed by the body, so consider waiting that long before breastfeeding your baby. It may not feel like the spontaneous Aperol Spritz you used to quaff, but by being clever with the timings of feeds, you can still enjoy a drink.
- Eating with your drink means that it is absorbed more slowly, so it can take longer for the alcohol to get metabolised and eliminated. This should be taken into consideration when timing your feeds.
- On average, it is estimated that alcohol levels in breast milk peak within 30–60 minutes after consumption, which means it doesn't go into the blood and breast milk straight away. You can, of course, feed your baby immediately before drinking, or if you wanted to maximise your time, you could even feed whilst you are sipping on a glass of wine (but be prepared for the ignorant, judgemental side-eye looks you'll get from other punters at the bar), and they are unlikely to be affected by that glass, providing the feed doesn't last more than 30 minutes. You could then feed your baby again, should they need it, a minimum of 2 hours later, thus still managing regular feeds.
- If you are planning to drink more than one standard drink, consider expressing first and feeding your baby with that milk. Please note that 'pump and dump' does not work. This term refers to expressing your milk and throwing it away. A myth developed that if you expressed your milk having been drinking alcohol, you could lessen the alcohol

content in your milk and therefore feed your baby safely. However, we
know that the alcohol level in breast milk is equivalent to the alcohol
level in a mother's bloodstream, so, even with pumping and dumping,
your breast milk continues to contain alcohol for as long as alcohol is
in your bloodstream. You may still choose to pump and dump if you
want to maintain your milk supply by frequently expressing, or if your
breasts have become uncomfortable, or you want to avoid mastitis or
engorgement. However, I am often loath to pour that precious nectar
down the sink, so I suggest holding onto the milk and doing a
'Cleopatra', by using it in the bath. That might sound strange, but she
was onto something. Due to its antimicrobial properties and its many
nutrients and minerals, it can be nourishing, and studies have shown
breast milk is as effective as 1 per cent hydrocortisone (steroid cream)
at managing mild to moderate eczema and nappy rash[161].

The concerns around drinking excess alcohol are that it could be damaging to your baby's development. It can affect their sleep patterns, motor skills and cognitive development. Babies were found to have less active and total sleep and their REM cycles were also disrupted. However, there is little research on the effects of small amounts of regular or long-term alcohol on a baby's development.

It has also been found that babies drink less milk when their mother has been drinking alcohol, by up to 20–23 per cent[162], but it has been observed that they compensate for this by drinking more after, so there is unlikely to be any long-term issue with feeding if it's the occasional drink. Alcohol may also impair your own judgement and your ability to safely care for your baby. I will go on to discuss safe sleeping, but this is a reminder not to co-sleep if you have been drinking alcohol, as this can increase the risk of SIDS. It's an obvious point, but if you are planning a big night, make sure there is a responsible adult around to look after your baby.

Furthermore, if you are only just establishing your milk flow or have had any difficulties with your milk production, alcohol can affect your milk ejection reflex and, more chronically, can decrease milk production. Whilst one drink is unlikely to affect it, to avoid any impact on your milk supply, you may want to wait until breastfeeding is well established first, usually by the time your baby is 6–8 weeks old.

Ultimately, there are already so many obstacles when it comes to the continuation of breastfeeding, that I would like the occasional alcoholic beverage not to be one of them. Given the myriad benefits of breast-feeding, I will leave you with the comforting words of the NHS: 'Alcohol consumed occasionally in low or moderate amounts is unlikely to harm your baby'[163, 164].

CAFFEINE AND BREASTFEEDING BE PREPARED

Whilst pregnant, you are advised to limit your caffeine intake to 200mg a day, and sadly this restriction continues in breastfeeding. This feels pretty cruel when you have been woken every hour for a feed, nappy change or general disgruntlement. However, the reason is because caffeine can be transferred to your baby through your breast milk, and they are less able to process it, potentially making them more restless and keeping them awake. This is of particular pertinence when they are under 6 months old (i.e. the timeframe when you are most in need of the caffeine!). I gave up caffeine totally when pregnant with Harris and, because he was such a poor sleeper, I just ended up continuing on my decaffeinated/herbal crusade even after, in case it would be further detrimental to his sleep. I've actually quite enjoyed being caffeine-free (aside from chocolate, I'd be insane to give that up too) and non-reliant on stimulants, and I certainly don't miss those post-Nero palpitations. I'm not saying caffeine-free is necessary, and it's not for everyone, but it's also not the worst outcome of pregnancy and breastfeeding.

BREAST MILK STORAGE BABY'S HERE

Once expressed, storing breast milk properly is important in maintaining the nutritional value of the milk as well as its safety for your baby. Wash your hands thoroughly before expressing and handling breast milk and use storage bags or bottles specifically designed for storing it. They tend to have a label on them so you can write the date of expressing. It creates less waste of that precious fluid if you store the milk in small quantities rather than filling up each storage bag to the max.

Storage	Fresh expressed breast milk	Thawed, previously frozen breast milk
Room temp (19–22°C)	4–6 hours (literature varies)	Discard
Cooler with ice packs (0–4°C)	24 hours	Discard
Fridge (0–4°C)	8 days	24 hours
Fridge (>4°C)	3 days	24 hours
Ice compartment of fridge	2 weeks	Do not re-freeze, discard
Freezer (-18°C)	6 months	Do not re-freeze, discard

If you are unsure of the temperature of your fridge, then buy a fridge thermometer, or assume it is >4°C. The milk should be stored towards the back of the fridge, not in the door, which can have higher and more variable temperatures, and make sure it is away from any raw/uncooked products like meat and eggs. You can give expressed milk straight from the fridge without the need to heat it up if your baby doesn't mind cold milk, otherwise you can heat it under a warm tap or in a jug of warm water. Alternatively, you can also buy machines that will warm milk to the desired temperature.

If you are thawing frozen breast milk, it is best to do so slowly in the fridge and use it within 24 hours. However, if you need to use it immediately, you can defrost it by putting it in a jug of warm water or holding it under running warm water. Don't worry if it looks different once defrosted, it tends to just need a shake as it may have separated.

Irrespective of whether it was refrigerated or defrosted, once your baby tucks into it, the breast milk must be drunk within an hour, and anything left over past that time should be discarded.

TROUBLESHOOTING – WHAT CAN GO WRONG
BABY'S HERE

Breastfeeding experiences vary significantly, with some having a smooth and easy ride and others hitting obstacles on the way. Many of the challenges can be overcome with the right knowledge and support, but when you're tired, emotional and in pain, it's not always easy to see the light at the end of the tunnel. It goes without saying that this trouble-shooting tool should not be used instead of seeking support from your midwife, health visitor, GP, lactation consultant, or anyone with the right experience, but it may just offer you a few tips to get you started whilst you're waiting for that support to arrive. In terms of breastfeeding knowledge, there is a significant variation in training and experience within healthcare professionals. Where some will offer sound, evidence-based advice and support, others may give biased or out-of-date information which can derail parents' breastfeeding experiences and journeys. It is important for a parent who is seeking support to ask the healthcare professional what training and qualifications they have. There is certainly a hierarchy of breastfeeding education, and those with the International Board Certified Lactation Consultant's (IBCLC's) credential is the highest-regarded professional qualification in breastfeeding knowledge and support, recognised worldwide.

HELP! MY NIPPLES ARE SORE

It is often said that breastfeeding shouldn't be painful. However, in the first couple of weeks of breastfeeding I found the soreness agonising. It felt like razorblades at the beginning of every feed. My latch was checked, Harris was checked for tongue-tie, I was assessed for thrush, my positioning was optimised, but none of these things helped.

Eventually the pain just went away by itself, and I never really knew what the cause was, but I assumed it was just hormonal tenderness. The following are common causes for nipple soreness:

Latch – if your baby is not latched on properly, not only do they not extract the milk effectively, but it also becomes painful for you. Whilst pain is the best sign that the latch isn't optimal, in some cases, a suboptimal latch can cause a 'lipstick'-shaped nipple. A poor latch can cause the nipple to taper at the end, similar to on a lippie. Go back to the section on how to establish breastfeeding (page 192) and try all the steps for an optimal latch one by one, remembering to ensure the baby's mouth covers a large portion of the areola and not just the nipple. Also, try the different positions, as you might find the baby is able to get a deeper latch when held in different ways.

Tongue-tie – this is a condition where the fold of tissue under the baby's tongue (the lingual frenulum) that connects the tongue to the bottom of the mouth is shorter or tighter than usual and therefore does not allow for the normal movement of the tongue and latching on properly. As the baby has restricted tongue movement, they may end up pinching the nipple between their tongue and hard palate, resulting in nipple pain. Other signs your baby might have tongue-tie can include poor weight gain, difficulty staying latched, feeding for long periods of time and, frequently, fussiness and seeming unsettled whilst feeding, and clicking noises while feeding. If you have any suspicions of tongue-tie, it should be examined by your healthcare provider, but you can have a look yourself too, and you might notice your baby's tongue doesn't lift or move from side to side easily and it can have a heart-shaped appearance when they stick it out. If tongue-tie is suspected you will be referred to a specialist for assessment and confirmation, and to determine whether a simple procedure is required. This surgical procedure involves cutting the tight frenulum to allow it to move more freely. Unfortunately, few healthcare providers are trained to assess for tongue-tie, and many confidently rule it out without explaining to the parents that they do not have the qualification to do so and without performing a comprehensive assessment. As such, if you have any concerns, you must ensure you are being signposted to the right place.

Thrush – this is a fungal infection, often referred to as candida, which can lead to nipple pain on breastfeeding, and it may also cause itchiness to your nipples.

It tends to occur when your nipples are cracked or dry. It can also affect the baby, with them developing white patches on their tongue or cheek. If this is the case, both mum and baby can be treated with antifungal medication. Interestingly, thrush tends to be over-diagnosed, and, if there is any doubt about the diagnosis, a swab can be taken of the mother's nipple and the baby's mouth to confirm thrush first. The symptoms of thrush are a sudden pain to both breasts/nipples after some weeks of pain-free breastfeeding. This pain comes on with every feed and can last up to an hour after the feed. It should not be diagnosed if it is only in one breast/nipple, or if the pain has been present since birth (so that you have never had any pain-free breastfeeding). Signs that your baby has thrush in their mouth are creamy/white patches on their tongue that do not rub off. There may also be a white gloss to their lips or tongue. Remember, milk can also make the tongue look white and this is more common in the first few weeks whilst establishing breastfeeding latch, whereas if your baby has tongue-tie they are less able to throw the milk to the back of the mouth, so instead it coats the tongue.

Nipple trauma – your nipples go through a lot whilst breastfeeding, and using incorrectly sized breast pumps or rough handling of your breasts can cause nipple trauma. A poor latch can also cause nipple damage and trauma. Treat them kindly, and ensure proper techniques when expressing and gentle handling when feeding.

Milk blister – this is a little small white blob that appears on the nipple. They tend to be caused by friction or your baby rubbing the nipple or compressing it against their hard palate, but can also be caused by a bit of skin blocking one of the nipple openings. They look so small and innocent, but they can really hurt – a bit like an inconspicuous blister on your foot! They tend to improve with readjusting the latch or position, but do not be tempted to pop it yourself as this can lead to infection.

Whilst addressing these potential causes, you can help improve the symptoms.

- Even though the evidence is sparse, I found using lanolin on my nipples really helped. Maybe it was simply the act of caring for yourself in an easily achievable way, the soothing moisturising or maybe it was just the barrier that it provided, but whatever the reason, that tube of yellow gloop stayed close by my side.

- If your nipple is very dry and cracked, in addition to an organic balm like lanolin you can also use a hydrogel dressing/pad to further protect the wound.
- Rubbing your own breast milk into your nipples offers antimicrobial benefits and works as a barrier against losing the natural moisture of the skin.
- Avoid retaining moisture on your nipples for long periods, as this can cause the softening of the skin and increase the risk of damage, it can also be a perfect environment for fungi to thrive. Let your nipples dry out after each feed before putting your bra back on, regularly change your breast pads and wear breathable cotton bras. Don't use a hairdryer to dry your nipples as this can cause further damage.
- Don't use soap on your breasts, as it can strip away our natural lubricants that protect our nipples. If you want to wash, try an emollient soap substitute, to avoid them drying out.
- It can be tempting to use a nipple shield or breast shell to create a barrier between your baby's mouth and your nipple to protect your sore nipples, but these may hinder your baby's latch and further propagate the issue.
- You may notice some improvement if you hand-express or pump for a few minutes before you feed to bring on a let-down, so your baby does not need to suckle so aggressively at the beginning of the feed.
- If you want to end a feeding session, break the latch gently by inserting a clean finger into the corner of your baby's mouth to break the suction. This will avoid further pulling and discomfort.
- Consider alternating feeds with breast pumps to give your nipples a break from an overzealous mouth. Though continued breastfeeding can actually help to promote healing because of the enzymatic action and healthy bacterial exchange from your baby's saliva. I know it feels like it will never heal, but your breast and nipple is a highly vascular area and it will heal, even with continued breastfeeding.

HELP! MY NIPPLES ARE BLEEDING

Bloody discharge can occur in up to 20 per cent of pregnant women or in the early postpartum period in breastfeeding women[165]. It is related to breast growth and increased blood flow as the breasts prepare to make milk. It tends to occur from both breasts and is usually self-limiting. However, when your nipples are cracked and sore they can also start to bleed. This can be as a result of postpartum skin changes, cracked nipples, mastitis and trauma. When there is no pain associated with the bleeding, it may be related to an uncommon condition called rusty pipe syndrome. It is given this name as the milk can have a colour similar to the dirty water that comes out of a rusty pipe, due to the colostrum mixing with a small amount of blood. It occurs as a result of increased blood flow to the delicate network of capillaries in the breasts. In most cases this spontaneously resolves within a week after the onset of breast-feeding and does not need any intervention.

It is important to address any of the possible underlying causes, which can be done by following the Help! My nipples are sore, and Help! My breasts are sore sections, but you can continue to breastfeed even when bleeding. Your baby might swallow a small amount of the blood whilst they feed, which can then show up as bright red blood in their posset or as darker blood in their stool. This might look alarming, but these small volumes are not harmful to your baby. It may, however, change the taste of the milk, so you might find your baby fussing over feeds more. Of course, if your baby is presenting with blood in their stool or vomit without you having bleeding nipples, you must consult your doctor. Furthermore, if you cannot identify where the bleeding is coming from, you should also discuss this with your doctor. Whilst it is considered safe to continue breastfeeding despite bleeding, the exception would be if you have an infection that can be transferred through blood, for example HIV or hepatitis.

HELP! MY BABY WON'T LATCH

You imagine this to be the most simple task – baby, nipple, attach. But breastfeeding is a learned process that often requires practice and does not necessarily come naturally to every mother and baby.

In the first instance, ensure that you and your baby are in a comfortable position, and use pillows if that helps. If one position isn't working for you, try others (see find the right position, page 193 to see the options) to get the correct alignment of your baby's mouth and your breast. It can be difficult for your baby to tilt their heads back and swallow easily if their head and neck are twisted, or their neck and shoulders aren't supported. Avoid supporting the head too rigidly at the back, though, as this may prevent your baby being able to tilt it backwards, which means they can't get a full mouthful and the nipple would just hit the hard roof of the mouth rather than the soft palate at the back.

Ensure you follow the steps to help your baby latch. It's tempting when you are tired and fed up to just lean your breast forward into their mouth and speed up the process, but it is important in this case that Mohammad comes to the mountain and you bring your baby to the breast to let them latch themselves.

You might find that prepping beforehand can help. Skin-to-skin contact before feeding may encourage you both to relax into it and encourage your baby's natural instinct to latch. Gently massaging your breasts before feeding may also stimulate the let-down reflex, which may help the process. You could even express a small amount of milk before feeding to help soften the breast and make it easier for the baby to latch. This is particularly relevant if your breasts are engorged or your nipples are flat or inverted.

If you have tried getting your baby in a perfect alignment to latch when they are screaming and headbutting your boob, you will know that a fussy, hungry, agitated baby is going to be harder to breastfeed. Watch out for those hunger cues and try to feed them before they get to that stage. If they are already at that stage, try to calm them down before getting them to latch on. You can consider rocking, swaddling or feeding in dimmed, quiet rooms.

HELP! I'M NOT MAKING ENOUGH MILK

One of the reasons breastfeeding can be difficult is the worry that you are not enough for your baby. As opposed to bottle feeding, you have no idea how much milk they are taking in, and managing this unknown can kick up a lot of anxiety and fears of inadequacy. Concerns about not producing enough breast milk is one of the main reasons cited as to why mothers move on from exclusively breastfeeding to mixed feeds. There are a number of signs to look for to determine whether your baby is getting enough milk:

Weight – it is normal in the first 2 weeks for your baby to lose weight, but, after this point, steady weight gain is a positive indicator that they are getting enough milk.

Nappies – observe your baby's poo and wee. After the initial meconium poos, you should note more frequent yellow poos, at least twice daily, in a baby aged 4 days to 6 weeks, but often more. In the first couple of days, there are likely only to be two or three wet nappies, but this should increase daily so that by the first week, your baby should be producing at least six wet nappies a day.

Noises – check they are making rhythmic sucking and swallowing sounds whilst breastfeeding. You should also see them swallowing with a slow, rhythmic jaw movement seen in front of the ear.

Satisfaction – they should look relaxed and calm throughout the feed, come off the breast on their own and appear content and satisfied after or they may fall asleep (though if your baby is a newborn, falling asleep at your breast is not on its own a reliable sign of satiety). They may do non-nutritive sucks which look like faster fluttery sucks once they have finished their feeds, or they may refuse the breast when re-offered or when offered the other breast. They should be alert when they are awake, being responsive and engaging with their surroundings.

Your breasts – if your breasts are softer after a feed, the chances are there is enough going into your baby, and remember that there is a feedback system with your breasts, so the more they feed, the more milk you produce. Check your nipples are the same shape and colour pre- and post-feeds to suggest the latch is adequate, and look for milk dripping from the other breast. In the first few days after delivery, adequate breastfeeding can increase your womb contractions and your lochia flow.

If you have concerns that you aren't producing enough milk, there are a number of things you can do to help rectify this and 'boost' your supply:

- This comes up time and time again, but check for the proper latch and optimise your position as this can affect how well your baby is able to drink and therefore lead to a decreased supply. Ask your midwife or health visitor to refer you for breastfeeding support – this may be at a drop-in centre or a specialist feeding team who comes to your home, they can observe you breastfeeding to make sure there is nothing else that can be done to improve it.

- Unless advised by your healthcare professional, avoid introducing bottles of formula until breastfeeding is well established. This is simply because, ideally, you want to increase the frequency and duration of your feeds to stimulate more milk production, rather than risk decrease it by supplementing the feeds. You can even help boost your supply by expressing after feeds.

- Feed on demand, which means as often and for as long as they want. Always offer both breasts when feeding, and alternate which breast you start with. To remember which I started with on the last feed, I would always wear a scrunchie around the corresponding hand.

- Avoid the use of dummies until breastfeeding is established. This is because babies have a natural instinct to suckle, and by using a dummy they may satisfy this need without actually feeding. In some babies it is also thought that dummies might cause nipple confusion, where they find it difficult to differentiate between the real nipple and the dummy, affecting their ability to latch and therefore affecting milk supply. Breastfeeding is usually well established by 4 weeks, and it is advised to wait until this point before introducing a dummy.

- Power pumping is a technique that is meant to mimic cluster feeding and promote increased milk production. It is not first-line advice, but it involves pumping frequently for short periods of time. An example of a power-pumping schedule can be expressing for 15 minutes, then taking a 30-minute break and repeating for 4 hours. You should aim to do this for three consecutive days for the best effect. Power pumping does not replace regular pumping or feeding, it is in addition to your normal routine. The key to milk supply is simply frequent and efficient milk removal, so the primary advice is still to make sure your baby is feeding well and often.

- You may find your baby squeezing at your breasts whilst they feed. Gentle compressions can help improve milk flow, so try massaging the breasts whilst feeding to help empty the breasts more effectively. It can help to massage your breast with a hand action that rolls the knuckles downwards over the breast, beginning at the top of the breast and working towards the areola, gradually going over the whole breast. Warm compresses on the breast prior to a feed may also improve milk flow.
- Ensure you are eating and drinking well, to support your milk production. Limit alcohol consumption, which can interfere with production.
- You use up a lot of water during milk production, equating to roughly 700ml per day at 8 weeks postpartum.[166] Whilst there is no hard and fast rule about exactly how much extra water you should drink whilst breastfeeding and it has not been well studied, it is important to be mindful of this potential fluid deficit. I always felt intensely thirsty every time I breastfed, and when he drank I drank. I would recommend always having a bottle of water to hand, and drinking whenever you feel thirsty to meet the needs of yourself and your breastfeeding baby.

There are lots of reported foods that claim to help boost milk production, which are known as galactagogues, though most mothers do not need herbal or medicinal treatments:

Oatmeal – there is no evidence that oatmeal boosts your milk supply directly[167], however, lots of mothers swear by it and, fighting its corner, it has a number of key nutrients in it that are healthy for mother and baby and can be really tasty. So if you feel it works for you, go for it.

Fenugreek – this has been used for centuries, though there are only a limited number of published studies to support the use of fenugreek in increasing milk supply and they are of poor quality[168]. It's generally considered safe and fairly well tolerated, but there are some reported gastrointestinal side-effects, and it is not advised in some health conditions like low blood pressure, insulin-controlled diabetes and clotting disorders.[169]

Fennel – the studies supporting its use are few and of low to moderate quality, so it would be difficult to state there is robust evidence that fennel increases milk supply[170]. However, as with oatmeal and fenugreek, there is plenty of anecdotal 'evidence'.

Easier said than done, but stress and fatigue can have a negative impact on milk production, so where possible try to get enough sleep by seeking support from partners, friends and family, and practise relaxation techniques to help you manage stress.

HELP! I'M MAKING TOO MUCH MILK

Whilst your body regulates how much milk to make, you can start to look like Dolly Parton – which can be very uncomfortable. If your baby can't fully drain the tense breast, it can also result in blocked ducts or mastitis. Other signs that you might have oversupply include leaking. It is normal for all breasts to leak milk, but if it is excessive, or continues to occur despite your baby having just fed, it may be an indicator. Your baby may also find it difficult to drink from your breasts when they are significantly full and they may cry, seem restless, struggle and try to pull off the breast whilst they feed. Or they may clamp down on the nipple in an attempt to slow down the flow of milk, which can be uncomfortable for you. Some babies will cough and splutter, or swallow a lot of air, resulting in being uncomfortable and gassy or having large possets. Posseting is a term that is only ever used in the parenting realm, and until you are a parent, it has little relevance in your life. It is simply the milky spit up that your baby brings up during or after a feed, and is the reason why you need to invest in a neverending supply of muslins to wipe it all up.

One way to help your baby with the fast flow is to practise the laid-back feeding position (see positions, page 193) as it gives your baby a bit more control. They are able to freely lift up their heads if they need a break.

The best way to regulate your supply is to feed on demand and produce the amount of milk that matches your baby's needs. Wear nursing pads to help stay dry when leaking, and if you need to express in between feeds to relieve the pressure, try to limit the duration as much as possible, as the more you remove the more you produce.

There is a technique known as block feeding that can be tried to reduce your milk supply. It involves feeding your baby on demand for a specified amount of time (often suggested as 4 hours initially, but it can be increased in incremental 2 hours until the desired effect is achieved) exclusively from one breast. After that block of time, you switch to the other breast for the next feeding block, and you continue alternating in this way. The aim of block feeding is to allow the whey protein in milk to build up by not being removed, sending feedback to slow down milk production.. Another similar technique also adds in full drainage before the block feeding. This means that you fully express your breast milk before beginning the block-feeding technique. There are risks to employing both of these techniques, including engorgement, mastitis and issues with nutritional intake for the baby, so they should be recommended and overseen by a lactation consultant who can ensure you have an individualised plan and that your baby's weight is closely monitored during this intervention.

HELP! MY BABY WON'T STOP FEEDING

It's hard not to question, well, everything when it comes to breastfeeding. Why is he so hungry? Am I producing enough milk? My boobs feel so empty, there can't be anything left in them for him?! Remember that your boobs are not just milk storage units, they make the milk too and do so fairly constantly, so even when it feels like your baby has been feeding incessantly and there cannot possibly be any more milk left in these flagging pancakes, be reassured there is a constant stream and they are never truly empty. Providing your baby is growing and thriving, pooing, weeing and happy (for the most part!) then you don't need to question your supply. The likelihood in this situation is that your baby has started cluster feeding. This is when your baby starts to feed more frequently in a condensed period of time. It usually coincides with a growth spurt, so your baby is seeking additional nutrition to support the spurt, but it can also happen if they just didn't feed enough before, they had a longer sleep, or they are simply craving more comfort. Whilst cluster feeding is totally normal, it is fair to say it is also totally exhausting for you. Most cluster feeds usually only last 2–7 days, so stick with it, and take that leap of faith that it will be ok. In the interim, stay hydrated, look after your nipples, sleep when you can, eat well and find a good box set to watch.

HELP! MY BREASTS ARE SORE

To manage sore breasts, it is usually necessary to understand the underlying cause. It may be related to a poor latch, engorgement/oversupply or thrush. We have addressed all of these areas in the troubleshooting above. Mastitis is another cause of breast pain. It is the inflammation of the breast tissue that can occur when there is a blockage in the milk ducts. This may be as a result of a poor latch, missed feeds, favouring one breast for feeds over the other, or even tight clothing. Where there is milk stasis, it can also allow bacteria to build up and cause an infection. The symptoms of mastitis include breast pain, redness (which may not be obvious in darker skin tones) and swelling. Your breast can be hot and painful to touch, and you may note a lump or hard area on it. You may also develop flu-like symptoms.

To treat mastitis you should:

- Try to clear the blocked ducts by continuing to feed your baby, and do so regularly to avoid them becoming overfull. It may feel counterintuitive to give yourself more pain, but do feed from the affected side first so that your baby is more likely to drain it. In 2022 the guidance on the management of mastitis was revised and it steered away from overfeeding from the affected breast or 'pumping to empty', as this could perpetuate a cycle of hyperlactation which may be a risk factor for worsening swelling and inflammation[171]. So simply continue to feed from the breast as normal.
- Recheck your baby's latch and position to ensure they are feeding optimally.
- Avoid wearing tight clothing and bras that might restrict the milk flow.
- You may find that a warm compress and warm bath will also help improve the milk flow. Massaging the breast may help to reduce the

pain but it should no longer be recommended as standard care due to the risk of trauma. Deep massage can cause increased inflammation, swelling and injury to the delicate blood vessels, so it is important that if you undertake any massage it is gentle, like the compressions you would do during a breast pump or hand expression. Avoid the use of electric toothbrushes and other commercial vibrating or massaging devices.

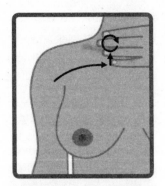

- The manual lymphatic drainage technique with light sweeping of the skin is more successful than deep tissue massage. The technique involves using a very gentle touch to the skin 'like petting a cat', when making 10 small circles with your fingertips between your internal jugular and subclavian vein (shown in images on right). Then do a further 10 circles in your armpit, after which you can continue with a light touch massage from your nipple in the direction of your collar bone (clavicle) and armpit[172].

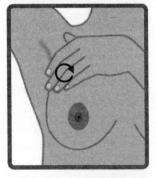

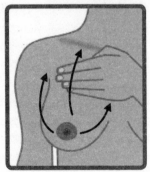

I had mastitis twice, both relating to times I had missed a feed, and I remember just sitting in a hot bath, gently rubbing my boob over and over again, with tears streaming down. It was not a pretty sight. On one of the occasions I needed antibiotics, on the other I gently massaged the blocked duct and managed to avoid medication.

If you are struggling with breast pain you can take paracetamol and ibuprofen, which also act as anti-inflammatories to relieve the swelling.

A cold compress can be used to relieve the pain, as can cold cabbage leaves! I know this is usually found in the vegetable drawer of your fridge rather than atop your cleavage, however, it has long been used as a home remedy to relieve breast pain. The mechanism of action is not fully understood but a cabbage leaf (with the hard stem removed for comfort) perfectly conforms to the shape of your breast, which might offer gentle support and a cold compress effect. The phytochemicals that the cabbage contains may also have anti-inflammatory properties to help reduce pain and inflammation.

If your symptoms are not getting better with these interventions, your GP may prescribe you antibiotics. Whilst a small amount of this medication goes into the breast milk, it is safe to take whilst breastfeeding, though it may make your baby have runnier poo or be a bit more irritable than normal.

HELP! I'M RETURNING TO WORK

I found returning to work exhilarating and terrifying in equal measures. I was desperate to be able to sit down at a desk, have a hot cup of coffee and do a wee without two huge eyes staring up at me, unblinking. However, I was also devastated about leaving the most precious thing I had ever made in the hands of someone else. I took a photo of the last morning I breastfed Harris before starting work, and at the time I thought it was a sweet photo, but when I look back at it, I had a real sadness in my eyes. I was scared that it might mean the premature end to my breastfeeding journey, that it would change our relationship, and that he would realise he didn't really need me that much after all. If only at the time I had the retrospect of knowing I would still be feeding him years later, actively trying to prize the boobie monster off me. But I totally understand the fear of wondering how you are going to cope with work and breastfeeding. I had a number of embarrassing or traumatic occasions at work when I was in the middle of pumping and a colleague would knock on the door, or worse, just walk in. Or when there was a queue building up behind me in the staff kitchen to use the microwave whilst I sterilised my pumping equipment. Or having nowhere to store my pumped breast milk, so it was just sitting in the staff fridge next to someone's tuna salad, or in a cool pack in my room, eternally fearing it will 'go off'.

At the time I thought I was a burden to everyone, I didn't want to make a fuss, I just wanted to get back to work and be 'normal' in my primarily male workspace. If I could do it all again, I would have reminded myself that what I was doing was nothing to be embarrassed about, that it was normal and, actually, it was better than normal, it was incredible. I was working and feeding my child.

Interestingly, in the UK there is no obligation for employers to provide a separate private environment for safely expressing and storing milk. The Health and Safety Executive (HSE) recommends that it is 'good practice for employers to provide a private, healthy and safe environment for breastfeeding mothers to express and store milk. The toilets are not a suitable place to express breast milk.' Workplace regulations do, however, require employers to provide suitable facilities where breastfeeding mothers can rest. Whilst a little rest is something we all appreciate, I'm sure, breastfeeding facilities would be better. The HSE advice is that this area to rest should be hygienic and private so that you can express yourself if you choose to, and should include somewhere to store your milk[173]. My advice would be to put in writing to your employer that you will be breastfeeding on your return to work, and the employer must then conduct a specific risk assessment.

Depending on when you return to work, it may even be that you do not need to express milk.

HELP! I CAN'T BREASTFEED IN PUBLIC

For many, breastfeeding in public is an entirely natural and normal way to nourish your baby, but others can feel uncomfortable or hold negative perceptions. This may be due to societal norms, public attitudes and cultural beliefs. Or it may be the fear of judgement or criticism from others that discourage breastfeeding mothers to nurse in public.

In an ideal world it would be great to find comfortable, private spaces to breastfeed that make us feel less exposed, but, from experience, these areas are few and far between. Ongoing public health campaigns and initiatives to promote and normalise breastfeeding go some way, as do supportive friends, family and groups to provide accepting environments. But, until policies and legislation to protect the rights of breastfeeding mothers are more fully advocated, if you want to avoid being chained to your house, it is helpful to find ways to overcome these barriers.

Firstly, I would start from within. You have every right to breastfeed in public, so be confident and self-assured in your decision to do so. Perhaps sit in front of a mirror at home to try to become more comfortable with it. You might find some positions are more comfortable and discreet. If you feel you need added privacy, carry a breastfeeding cover with you, and choose breastfeeding-friendly bras and tops that allow for more less-awkward access. They also just tend to be easier as you're not having to remove an entire dress in the middle of a cafe.

If you do receive any negative judgement, have a response ready in your arsenal to assertively educate the ignoramuses about the importance and normalcy of breastfeeding, reminding them that there are laws that protect a mother's right to breastfeed in public.

You will also find that hanging out with other mothers who feel more comfortable breastfeeding in public can offer a huge amount of encouragement for you. You feel so much more undefeatable when you are feeding en masse.

On a wider scale, we should all be doing our best as mothers to advocate for breastfeeding-friendly environments, promoting awareness and helping to remove any barriers created to support breastfeeding mothers in public.

Breastfeeding is a wondrous challenge. Having been through the chaotic newborn stage, the routined infant stage, the uncertain weaning stage, and through the other end with an extended toddler feeding stage, I could say that I am well versed in all things milk production, but the truth is I am probably still as flummoxed as everyone at the beginning of their journeys because every stage brings its own set of hoops to jump through.

Sometimes feeling exasperated and fed up, other times so grateful I have this tool, I've used breastfeeding to troubleshoot every issue I've had with my child. Tired? Breastfeed. Hungry? Breastfeed. Vaccinations? Breastfeed. Got an ouchie? Breastfeed. On a flight? Breastfeed. Ill? Breastfeed. Needing connection? Breastfeed. Hot? Breastfeed. Cold? Breastfeed. I've whacked out my boobs on so many occasions just to give myself the time to record a podcast, or take an important call, whether or not Harris needed or wanted a feed! These two fleshy, saggy, milk-laden blobs of adipose have saved my bacon on a number of occasions. I think at times I would have had to be a far more creative and patient parent if I didn't breastfeed, as I would have needed to find other ways to manage all these common kiddie issues. That being said, I have no doubt that had I not been able to, or chose not to breastfeed, my love and bond for my boy would be exactly the same.

FORMULA FEEDING `BABY'S HERE`

Should you be unable to, or choose not to, breastfeed, you will bottle feed your child with formula milk. This may be exclusively or you may do mixed feeds (formula and breast). Much of the advice around feeding your baby remains the same in terms of paying attention to your baby's cues, feeding them responsively, finding quiet and calming environments for them to feed in and burping them after. You should also take the opportunity, when possible, to practise skin-to-skin contact when feeding to promote bonding and a sense of security. Bottle feeding still remains an important time for love, comfort and connection, and is not just about nourishment.

WHICH FORMULA MILK SHOULD YOU CHOOSE?

There are many variants of formula available. First infant formula is the first milk you should offer your newborn. It has whey (rather than casein) protein in it, which is easier for newborns to digest. They can continue to drink this throughout their first year, and there is no evidence to suggest any benefit to switching them to the Follow-on formula after six months[174]. First infant formula most commonly is made from cow's milk, but there is also goat's milk available, and they have the same nutritional standards as each other.

There are other types of formulas available, depending on the specific needs of your child.

Hungry formula – contains more casein than whey, which takes them longer to digest.

Anti-reflux formula – thickened with the aim to reduce reflux, suitable under medical supervision.

Comfort formula – this has partly broken-down proteins to make it easier to digest in babies with digestive problems like colic and constipation, however, there is no evidence for this.

Lactose-free formula – this is suitable, under medical supervision, for babies who have lactose intolerance or issues digesting lactose, a natural sugar found in milk.

Hypoallergenic formula – this has fully broken-down proteins, required if your baby has been diagnosed with CMPA (see page 262).

Soya formula – this is made from soya beans and can be offered only after 6 months under medical supervision.

If you have concerns that your child may need one of these special types of formulas, it would be best to discuss it with your midwife, health visitor or GP. However, the NHS also has a website to guide you further through the world of formula.[175]

HOW TO PREPARE FORMULA FEEDS SAFELY

Formula comes in two forms, a dry powder that you mix with water and ready mixed liquid. The latter is more convenient, but also more expensive and has a shorter shelf life once opened.

It is important to follow the preparation instructions on the container carefully as they can vary in terms of water and formula measurements. The NHS has provided a step-by-step guide[176]:

1. Fill the kettle with at least 1 litre of fresh tap water (do not use water that has been boiled before).
2. Boil the water. Then leave the water to cool for no more than 30 minutes, so that it remains at a temperature of at least 70°C.
3. Clean and disinfect the surface you are going to use.
4. It's important that you wash your hands.
5. If you are using a cold-water steriliser, shake off any excess solution from the bottle and the teat, or rinse them with cooled boiled water from the kettle (not tap water).
6. Stand the bottle on the cleaned, disinfected surface.
7. Follow the manufacturer's instructions and pour the amount of water you need from the kettle into the bottle. Double-check that the water level is correct. Always put the water in the bottle first, while it is still hot, before adding the powdered formula.
8. Loosely fill the scoop with formula powder, according to the manufacturer's instructions, then level it using either the flat edge of a clean, dry knife or the leveller provided. Different tins of formula come with different scoops. Make sure you only use the scoop that comes with the formula.
9. Holding the edge of the teat, put it into the retaining ring, check it is secure, then screw the ring onto the bottle.
10. Cover the teat with the cap and shake the bottle until the powder is dissolved.
11. It's important to cool the formula so it's not too hot to drink. Do this by holding the bottle (with the lid on) under cold running water.
12. Test the temperature of the formula on the inside of your wrist before giving it to your baby. It should be body temperature, which means it should feel warm or cool, but not hot.
13. If there is any made-up formula left in the bottle after a feed, throw it away.

HOW TO CHOOSE WHICH BOTTLES AND NIPPLES TO USE

There are many varieties of bottles and nipples available, all with different features, sizes, shapes, materials and flow rates.

Bottles come in two sizes – 150ml and 250ml – and for a newborn the smaller size will suffice. As they get older and hungrier you can move on to the larger bottle size. There are 'normal' bottles and wide-necked bottles that can be easier to fill and clean. You can also buy anti-colic bottles, which are designed to reduce the amount of air swallowed, though there is no independent research into whether these claims are substantiated. Always check the bottles for damage and cracks and replace them if needed.

Teats come in silicone or latex and in varying shapes. Newborns tend to need slower-flow nipples (they have fewer holes in them) to prevent choking, and give them better control over how they feed, but as they grow older they may need a medium or fast flow to help satisfy their growing appetite. The teats can get damaged easily, especially when the little teeth start to come through, so check them regularly. Silicone teats tend to be more robust than latex ones.

STERILISING AND CLEANING BOTTLES

Babies under 1 year must have their bottles and teats sterilised before using them. This is because harmful bacteria can build up, and with their immature immune systems babies are more vulnerable and could become ill if they drank milk contaminated with bacteria. After each feed, ensure they are washed thoroughly with specific bottlebrushes in warm and soapy water, or if they are dishwasher safe they can be popped in there.

There are several ways you can sterilise your bottles (and other feeding and pumping equipment):

Boiling – the boiling point of water is 100°C and at this temperature, for 10 minutes, most bacteria are killed. It is a simple method, all you need to do is disassemble the bottles, put them in a large pot, cover them with water, bring them to a rolling boil and keep it in there for 10 minutes. Keep them covered and remove them only before needing them.

Steam – there are specialised sterilisers that use steam, which, like boiling, brings the temperature to a point that bacteria are killed. In general, you add water to the steriliser, put the bottles and teats facing down inside and either plug it

into the mains or put it in the microwave. Follow the manufacturer's
instructions.

Chemical – this uses chemical sterilising solutions and tablets mixed with cold
water. You would soak the items, fully submerged in the solution, for at least
30 minutes. Then rinse the bottles thoroughly with cooled boiled water.

UV – specialised UV sterilisers kill microorganisms by denaturing their cell
structure and genetic material. The items can be used straight out of the
steriliser. Latex teats, however, cannot be used in this.

HOW MUCH MILK SHOULD I GIVE?

The amount of formula that your baby will drink will vary depending
on their age, weight, growth rate and individual appetite. Newborn
babies have tiny stomachs, only needing small volumes of formula
initially, and they will be feeding frequently, usually 8–12 times over 24
hours. As they grow, they will be able to consume larger amounts at each
feed and perhaps have fewer feeds each day. From their first week until
they are 6 months old, it is often cited that they will usually take in
150–200ml/kg in 24 hours[177], but this can be highly variable. The WHO
simply recommends responsive feeding by putting as much as you want
in the bottle and letting the baby take as much as they want, whilst
observing for the cues of satiety, growth and wet nappies to ensure they
are getting enough. From 7 to 9 months, they will drink around 600ml
per day, and from 10 to 12 months they will drink around 400ml per
day. This is, of course, only a guideline, and by practising responsive
feeding you will learn your baby's individual requirements. Babies are
generally good at regulating their own intake, so if they seem full or
uninterested, take the bottle away and don't force them to finish it.

Stacey Zimmels, a speech and language therapist specialising in
paediatric feeding and swallowing and IBCLC, recommends the
following responsive approach to bottle feeding.

'All babies feed best when they are fed when THEY want or are ready to
feed. So be responsive to this. Offer the bottle to your baby when they show

their first hunger cues. Crying is a late hunger cue. Early hunger cues include stirring from sleep with head turning from side to side, mouth opening and closing, tongue moving and taking hands to mouth. Wait for your baby to open their mouth for the teat. You can encourage this by rubbing the teat down from their nose to the mouth and dripping drops of milk on their lips. Offer pauses during feeding and stop the feed when your baby stops sucking and is showing signs that they have had enough.'

Common issues she gets asked in her work about bottle feeding include the following:

My baby is drinking more/less than it says on the tin.
As long as your baby is growing well and there are no medical concerns, it is fine to follow your baby's lead with volumes. The guideline volumes are an average and it is important to remember that every baby is different. Your baby may be bigger/smaller so need more/less, they may drink little and often or large amounts less often. This variability is normal too.

My baby never finishes a bottle.
As above, as long as your baby is growing well and there are no medical concerns, this is fine. Some babies feed little and often, especially newborns as their tummies are small.

My baby is now drinking less than before.
It's normal for milk volumes to fluctuate day to day. Your baby may drink more during a growth spurt, for example. It is also possible that your baby drinks larger volumes in the first few months when growth rate is very high and before their own appetite regulation is fully developed. Following this you may notice that the volumes reduce a little. If this happens it is very likely fine. Follow your baby's lead, don't force them to finish the bottle, watch for wet nappies and get their weight checked if you are concerned.
If you are at all concerned by their weight, seeming unsatisfied after feeds, or always being hungry, it is best to discuss this further with your health visitor or GP to rule out any underlying causes.

PACED FEEDING

This is a technique used when bottle feeding to mimic the natural flow and pace of breastfeeding, letting your baby control the flow of the milk. The aim is to ensure your baby is taking in an appropriate amount of milk and to reduce the risk of gas, posseting and colic. It can be a helpful method to use if you are breastfeeding but would like to introduce formula feeds too, as it utilises the same sucking techniques your baby is used to at the breast.

It requires you to hold your baby upright or slightly reclined, and gently touch the nipple/teat of the bottle to the baby's lip, allowing them to root and open their mouth naturally. Once they have latched on and started sucking, ensure that the bottle is tilted just enough so that the nipple has milk in it but is not completely full. This ensures the baby is actively sucking to allow the milk to flow, and it gives them the chance to take breaks during the feed. If they show signs of slowing down, you can help them pace the feed by partially removing the nipple or tilting the bottle down, offering a short break, then letting them suck on it again when they are ready.

FEEDING YOUR BABY: A TIRED MAMMA'S SUMMARY

Breast development and hormonal triggers: breast development begins during puberty, but the full ductal system necessary for breastfeeding matures during pregnancy due to hormonal changes. Oestrogen promotes the development of milk ducts, while progesterone supports the growth of lobules and alveoli, responsible for milk production. Milk travels from alveoli to the nipple through ducts that join together in the areola. During pregnancy, prolactin triggers colostrum production, but high levels of progesterone inhibit significant lactation until after birth.

Breast milk composition: breast milk contains all essential nutrients for the baby, including water, fats, carbohydrates, proteins, vitamins and minerals.

Colostrum, produced in the first days, has high immune components and nutrients. Transitional milk follows, becoming more calorific and higher in fat and lactose. Mature milk's composition remains fairly consistent but can vary based on factors like diet, hydration and nursing patterns.

Benefits of breastfeeding: breast milk provides optimal nutrition, immune support, reduced risk of chronic diseases, improved cognitive development and emotional connection for the baby. Benefits for the mother include emotional connection, postpartum recovery, reduced risk of chronic diseases and contraception. There are some challenges, including that it can be physically and emotionally demanding, impacting autonomy and lifestyle.

Alcohol and breastfeeding: alcohol does pass into breast milk. If you would like to consume alcohol there are ways to do it safely to minimise the baby's exposure, and potential effects on the baby's development.

Caffeine and breastfeeding: caffeine does pass into breast milk, which may have a potential impact on the baby's sleep patterns and restlessness.

Formula feeding: there are a number of types of formula to choose from, though most babies only require the standard age-appropriate formulations. This is also the case when purchasing bottles and teats. Appropriate sterilisation and cleaning techniques are imperative for safe feeding.

Paced feeding: this is a technique to mimic the natural flow and pace of breastfeeding while bottle feeding. It emphasises holding the baby upright, allowing them to control the feed's pace, and mimicking breastfeeding behaviours.

ISSUES ENCOUNTERED WHEN BREASTFEEDING

Sore nipples: this can be caused by factors such as poor latch, tongue tie, thrush, nipple trauma or milk blisters. Proper latch, positioning and gentle care of the nipples can help alleviate soreness. Using lanolin, rubbing breast milk on nipples, avoiding moisture retention and refraining from using soap on the breasts are additional strategies.

Baby won't latch: proper positioning and alignment are crucial for successful latching. Different positions should be tried to find the most comfortable and effective one. Skin-to-skin contact, breast massage and expressing a small amount of milk before feeding can encourage latching. Calming a fussy baby before attempting to latch is also suggested.

Low milk supply: signs that a baby is receiving enough milk include steady weight gain, appropriate nappy output, rhythmic sucking and swallowing sounds, and a content demeanour after feeding. To boost milk supply, ensuring proper latch, feeding on demand, avoiding formula supplementation, power pumping and practising relaxation techniques are recommended.

Oversupply of milk: oversupply can lead to breast discomfort, blocked ducts and other issues. Strategies to manage oversupply include feeding on demand, block feeding, wearing nursing pads and avoiding excessive pumping.

Continuous feeding: cluster feeding, often associated with growth spurts, can lead to frequent and prolonged feeding sessions. Staying hydrated, resting and nourishing oneself are important during this period.

Sore breasts: this can be caused by various factors, including poor latch, engorgement, mastitis, or blocked ducts. Proper latch, massaging, warm compresses and cabbage leaf application are ways to alleviate soreness. If necessary, over-the-counter pain relievers can be used, and antibiotics may be prescribed for mastitis.

Returning to work: balancing breastfeeding and work can be challenging. Expressing milk at work may require creating a supportive environment, including a designated space for pumping and storing milk. Communication with employers and advocating for breastfeeding accommodations is important.

Breastfeeding in public: overcoming discomfort with breastfeeding in public can involve building confidence, using discreet breastfeeding covers and wearing breastfeeding-friendly clothing. Advocacy for breastfeeding-friendly policies and normalising breastfeeding in society are key for addressing this challenge.

CHAPTER 8

SLEEP

Where do I even begin? Harris was broken. Or at least that's how I felt whenever I spoke to friends about their kids' sleep, or when I read about 'average' children's sleep. But Harris is an outlier, there are no two ways about it, he did not fit into the normal bell curve distribution of things. When the 'sleep experts' were saying he should be sleeping for 14 hours a night and having a 2-hour nap, he was sleeping for 9 hours and napping for 40 minutes. I spent a long time thinking I was doing something wrong, and I spent a lot of effort trying to 'fix' my deviant child.

I was looking at it all wrong. He was not at all broken, he's just a low sleep-need child, and being able to reflect on it all now, I knew there were no red flags, and I knew he would wake in the mornings and not look exhausted, so I should have trusted my instincts. But when you've been asked for the millionth time by well-meaning friends, colleagues and family, 'Does he sleep through the night yet?' it can be difficult not to question yourself. Eventually, I found a friend whose child had similar minimal sleep patterns to mine, and everything felt better again, I just needed to be reminded that I'm not the only parent out there struggling with sleep.

THE IMPORTANCE OF SLEEP BE PREPARED

One of the reasons we obsess so much about our baby's sleep is that we know how important it is for their development, and we are terrified that by not optimising their sleep as babies, we are denying them of their brilliant IQs and future Cambridge University degrees.

During sleep, the body releases growth hormones, which promote physical growth and brain development and allows our babies to consolidate the new skills and information they have acquired whilst awake. Their brains will have the chance to process and organise information, consolidating their memories and learning. It also helps in repairing tissues, rejuvenating the body and optimising the immune system. A well-rested baby will be more alert and focused, and they will be better equipped to handle the challenges of the day with more stable moods and less irritability.

NEWBORN SLEEP PATTERNS BE PREPARED

The million-pound question is, how much sleep is the right sleep? Sleep charts are a helpful guideline, but, as in my experience, there will be outliers who don't fit in the average sleep ranges, yet are still happy and thriving children. There are many unrealistic sleep expectations floating around in the new-parent world, so do not panic if your child doesn't fit into this neat little chart, but double-check for red flags.

Age	Average sleep in 24 hours	Average number of naps
0–3 months	14–17	Varies
4–11 months	12–15	3–4
1–2 years	11–14	1–2
3–5 years	10–13	0–1
6–13 years	9–11	0

The other bane of most new parents' existence are sleep cycles and wake windows. Most of you would not have spent much time caring about these terms in your own sleep before you had a baby, but suddenly, postnatally, they become primary features in your life.

A sleep cycle refers to the sleep stages that you go through whilst asleep and consists of non-rapid eye movement (NREM) and rapid eye movement (REM) sleep. An adult typically has a sleep cycle that lasts 90–110 minutes[178], but in a newborn it is shorter, typically lasting anywhere between 30 minutes and 70 minutes[179]. Newborns also spend more time than adults in REM sleep[180], which is important for their brain development.

Whilst older children and adults can wake between cycles, we are able to get ourselves back to sleep, often without even realising we have woken. However, newborns commonly need help and soothing to get them back to sleep between their cycles. This may take the form of feeding them back to sleep, rocking them, singing to them, patting them, or whatever works for you and your baby. I always just fed Harris back to sleep, as it was the path of least resistance and worked the fastest.

Wake windows refer to the time elapsed between sleep, and getting these right is thought to make falling asleep easier and helps to achieve restful sleep. The duration of wake windows varies depending on age, as newborns and infants need more naps and have shorter windows than older children. I got a little obsessed with wake windows with Harris in the first few months. I plotted his sleep in various apps and was beside myself when he went over the prescribed 45-minute wake window, and would immediately take him out for a walk in a sling to make him fall asleep. In all fairness to the little chap, when strapped onto me or my husband for a walk he almost always fell asleep quickly, but the concept of wake windows assumes that every baby of a certain age WILL become tired at the same time. However, our babies aren't all robots programmed to sleep in synchrony, and obsessing over the 'standard' or expected sleep cycles and wake windows can be a huge source of stress for parents. It can be useful to understand the different needs of a baby compared to an adult, but it is unlikely your baby will fit into the neat little boxes that some baby sleep educators imply they will.

The law of averages does mean that *some* babies will fit into the prescribed pattern, so if it works for you, then certainly use the wake windows as a guide to help you know when your baby will want to sleep. Whilst the length of wake windows for newborns can vary, they generally fit within the range of 45 minutes to 1.5 hours. This tends to extend by the time they are three to six months of age to 1.5 to 2.5 hours.

In those early days, I think I spent too much time watching the clock and not enough time looking at Harris' sleep cues and working out his unique sleep patterns. Babies may be non-verbal, but they are still constantly communicating with us, and your baby will often offer you cues that they are getting tired and need to sleep. It may be obvious, with yawning, a glazed-over expression or rubbing eyes, or it may be more subtle, with fussiness, irritability, moving their heads side to side, losing interest in toys, delayed responsiveness and crying.

RED FLAGS BE PREPARED

As discussed, variations in babies' sleep patterns are normal, but is there a point at which it isn't normal? There are some red flags that might indicate your baby's sleep is secondary to an underlying issue.

Excessive daytime sleepiness – some babies are low-sleep-need babies and are perfectly happy sleeping 20 per cent less than their peers. They are awake, alert and lively in the day. However, if your baby wakes and continues to be unhappy, irritable and sleepy, this may be a sign that they are not getting the amount of sleep they actually need.

Irregular or noisy breathing – if you notice your baby is breathing in an irregular pattern, for example, rapid, shallow breaths, or long pauses and gasping for air, it may indicate an underlying breathing disorder. Similarly, noisy breathing like snoring can also warrant further investigation.

Distress – a baby can cry for many reasons in the night, including hunger, discomfort and feeling hot or cold. However, if it is excessive or unexplained and they seem in distress, it could potentially be due to underlying issues.

Developmental concerns – if there are any other developmental concerns that you have for their age and developmental stage, sleep patterns may also be related to this.

Restless sleep – this can be more difficult to ascertain. Some babies just need help linking their sleep cycles, so they wake between each cycle signalling their need for support. This can be entirely normal – knackering, but normal. In others, frequent wake-ups may indicate a sleep disturbance.

I must reassure you that observing any of these red flags does not necessarily mean there is an underlying issue, and for the majority of babies there is probably nothing to worry about, but it is just a little prompt to seek a healthcare professional's advice. There are several underlying health conditions that the red flags could be indicative of, including, but not limited to:

Digestive issues – gastroesophageal reflux disease (GERD) is a disorder where the stomach acid refluxes back up into the oesophagus, resulting in discomfort. It can be particularly bad for a baby when they are laid flat as the acid does not have to work against gravity, thus disrupting sleep. Other symptoms can include excessive posseting, vomiting and crying. Allergies or sensitivities to foods can also trigger digestive issues that can disrupt sleep.

Respiratory conditions/sleep apnoea – conditions that affect breathing can affect sleep. This can include asthma, allergies, croup, bronchiolitis and sleep apnoea. Sleep apnoea in infants can be secondary to large tonsils or adenoids.

Pain – as with adults, pain can disrupt sleep in an infant. This may be related to ear or throat infections, gastrointestinal issues, teething and musculoskeletal problems.

Neurological conditions – conditions like epilepsy causing seizures can result in abnormal sleep patterns.

Iron deficiency – if your baby lacks sufficient iron, they may experience fatigue, weakness and difficulty sleeping. It may manifest in restless sleep with frequent wakings.

SLEEP PROGRESSION BABY'S HERE

There are a number of developmental milestones that can affect sleep, though the phrase often used is 'sleep regression'. I have an issue with this term as it implies a step backwards, a fault or a problem. But, in actual fact, these periods of time when sleep is affected are often because your baby is developmentally progressing.

Newborn sleep progression – as a newborn, there are a number of factors that affect sleep, including their immature circadian rhythm (not being able to tell day from night), everything being entirely new, frequent nappy changes in the night, needing fairly constant comfort and regular night feeds. Trying to help them regulate their circadian rhythm is the primary measure you can do to manage their sleep at this stage. This may mean keeping daytime sleep in bright environments and ensuring nighttime sleep is in the dark.

Four-month sleep progression – as they get older and become more sentient, wanting interaction and being more responsive, they may get more distracted by people, toys and sounds. This alertness may affect their ability to fall asleep as easily. Although the positive here is that their sleep cycle will start to lengthen and they will move from more REM sleep to deeper sleep. You can start to consider a vague bedtime routine so that they begin to grasp the concept of bedtime cues.

Six-month sleep progression – by the time they are 6 months old, most babies are able to sit, roll onto their backs and are babbling away. All this brain activity can lead to more vivid dreams and night wakings whilst they try to process new information, or increased restlessness. Your baby might start practising sitting up in their cot or rolling whilst they sleep, which can wake them up, or it might just stimulate them enough that all they want to do is practise this newfound skill rather than sleep. Your baby will also start eating solids, which may mean fewer night feeds and longer stretches of sleep, but not necessarily. Try keeping them stimulated and practising their new skills as much as they would like during the daytime so that they don't have as much of the need to do this at night. Ensure a regular peaceful and connecting bedtime routine that your baby can rely on for its sleep cues.

Eight–10-month sleep progression – here we get to the crawling stage (or bum shuffling, sliding, wriggling or whatever it might be!) and your baby just wants to explore everything. They have previously been entirely dependent on you to get them from A to B and suddenly they now have mobility. The urge to move and explore can impact how easily they will settle to sleep. They also develop separation anxiety at this stage, where they get scared that if you go away you might not actually come back. This might make them more clingy and resist being put to sleep. They may wake up more to check that you are still there and seek comfort and reassurance. Peekaboo type of games during the day can help reassure your baby that even if they cannot see you, you are always there, and you always come back.

Twelve-month sleep progression – babies tend to start walking or furniture walking and this motor-skill milestone can result in more active, restless sleep. Getting them outside and practising these skills in the fresh air allows them to explore all the fun new spaces at their disposal. They are able to communicate more, understand simple instructions and work on their own speech. Their brains are in over-drive, and it can feel overwhelming for them, so they may need more comfort and support than normal. This may all manifest in a change in sleep.

SIDS BE PREPARED

If you had asked me what my primary fear was about having a newborn, it wouldn't have been the sleep deprivation, breastfeeding, nappy changes or how it would affect my relationship, it was Sudden Infant Death Syndrome (SIDS). It is such a serious and unpredictable condition, that it made me feel so uneasy. Fortunately, it is rare, affecting 0.2–0.5 per 1,000 live births in most countries[181].

SIDS, sometimes also referred to as 'cot death' (though this term has largely been abandoned due to the suggestion that SIDS can only occur when the baby is asleep in its cot, which is not true), is the unexplained death of a baby, usually during sleep. It most commonly occurs in babies under 6 months old, and the cause is still not fully understood. It is thought that babies who die of SIDS are unable to respond appropriately to environmental stressors, and may have difficulty regulating their heart rate, breathing and temperature.

The risks of SIDS can be divided into intrinsic and extrinsic factors. Intrinsic factors are those that affect the vulnerability of the baby, increasing its susceptibility to the influence of extrinsic factors. Intrinsic factors tend to be ones that you cannot modify. Extrinsic factors are the physical stressors that are experienced by the baby that often relate to their environment. These can be modified.

INTRINSIC FACTORS

- Male sex – there is an increased incidence of SIDS in male babies (approximately 60 per cent male, 40 per cent female).
- Prematurity – before 37 weeks of pregnancy.
- Low birth weight – <2.49kg.
- Genetic polymorphisms – this is the presence of variant forms of a specific DNA sequence.
- Prenatal exposure to drugs – especially nicotine from cigarettes and alcohol.

EXTRINSIC FACTORS

- Sleep position – babies who are placed to sleep on their stomachs or sides.
- Sharing sleep surface – sharing an adult bed, sofa or armchair. The risk is even higher if the surface is soft, the adult is very tired or drowsy, the adult smokes, the baby is less than 4 months old, the adult is a caregiver other than the parent, the baby was premature or low birth weight, or the area includes unsafe items like pillows or blankets.
- Overheating – babies who are over-bundled, dressed in too many layers or the bedding is too warm for the room temperature. Babies are also more likely to overheat if they are placed on their stomachs to sleep.
- Soft bedding – sleeping on or under soft bedding. The risk of other sleep-related deaths from suffocation, entrapment (when a baby gets

trapped between two objects like the mattress and the wall) and strangulation is also higher.

- Inappropriate sleep surfaces – sleeping on an adult bed, couch or armchair alone, or with an adult, sibling or pet.
- Infant's face is covered.

There are a number of ways in which you can reduce the risk of SIDS:

- Put your baby down to sleep on their back.
- Share a room with your baby for the first 6 months. It is recommended they sleep close to your bed, but on their own separate, flat and clear surface designed for infants. They should remain in the same room as you for their daytime sleep too. Ensure they are not put to sleep near a radiator or sunny window, and any nearby blind cords or cables need to be secured away from your baby.
- Quit smoking.
- Do not sleep with your baby on a sofa or armchair.
- Do not sleep with your baby if you have been drinking alcohol, smoking, or have taken drugs or medication that could make you drowsy.
- Breastfeed if you can – breastfed babies are at lower risk for SIDS than formula-fed babies, but it doesn't have to be done for many months. Evidence suggests that breastfeeding for some time is more protective against SIDS than not at all[182] and that combination feeding offers some protection, albeit not as much as exclusive breastfeeding. It is thought that breastfeeding infers this advantage because of the physical process of suckling, which increases the baby's arousal thresholds, that is, they are easier to wake up. It also influences the mother's arousal, making it less likely you enter a deep sleep. Whilst breastfeeding, the baby's head will be more likely to be below the pillow and they are also less likely to be lying on their tummy. Furthermore, breastfeeding offers immunological benefits that reduce infection risks, which is one of the risk factors for SIDS.
- Dummies – babies who sleep with dummies are at lower risk of SIDS than those who do not[183].

CO-SLEEPING BE PREPARED

Co-sleeping is how I survived motherhood and lived to tell the tale. It is simply sleeping on the same surface as your baby. It gets a bad rep, mostly because of all the above fears around SIDS. Yes, the risks of SIDS are lower when your baby is on their own separate, firm surface. However, there is a huge difference between accidentally falling asleep with your baby and planning to co-sleep, and there is no differentiation in the statistics between the two when assessing the rates of SIDS. A 2022 report from the National Child Mortality Database showed that 52 per cent of SIDS in under 1-year-olds were when co-sleeping with an adult or older sibling. However, of those, 60 per cent had not been planned and 92 per cent were in hazardous circumstances[184]. This highlights the importance of meticulously planning the safety around co-sleeping.

Interestingly, rates of SIDS are lowest in countries where co-sleeping is the norm. This statistic does not account for other possible factors, like whether those countries also have lower rates of smoking or drinking alcohol, but I think it might be an interesting concept to consider whether the rates are lower because they aren't ashamed of co-sleeping, they talk about it openly, and therefore they are educated in how to limit the risks associated with it. We are told by so many different sources that the baby should sleep on their own surface, that even mentioning to a healthcare professional that you are co-sleeping can feel like you're failing, and you may choose not to tell anyone. But in keeping it hidden, you are risking not getting the right information on how to do it safely. The Lullaby Trust found on a recent survey during Safe Sleep Week 2023, that 9 in 10 parents co-sleep, but only 9 per cent had planned to do this before their baby was born[185]. So I think these statistics call for us to be honest with ourselves and each other about co-sleeping. It happens a lot, so even if you don't plan to co-sleep, expect that it probably will happen at some point, and make sure you know what to do to reduce the risks associated with co-sleeping.

- Remove any pillows and duvets that could cover your baby. I wear a long-sleeved top that keeps my top half warm enough and just have the duvet covering my lower legs.
- Tie your hair up. I have particularly long hair that could be a strangulation risk, so it gets scraped back into a low bun.
- Put any cables away. We all tend to charge our phones nearby overnight but the cable is a strangulation risk. Also, look out for curtain ties and blind cords.
- Don't place your baby in between yourself and your partner. It can increase the risk of suffocation or entrapment. As discussed above, a breastfeeding mother is less likely to enter a deep sleep, however, a partner may be less easily roused, so it would be sensible to keep the baby on the side of a breastfeeder, if that is an option. However, you also need to be mindful of how near the edge of the bed they are. We found a floor mattress the safest way to do this.
- Fill in any gaps. If there is a gap between the mattress and headboard or between the bed and the wall, your baby can get wedged in, so ensure these are filled. Ideally you would position a floor bed in the middle of the room, away from walls and other furniture, with space around it.
- Ensure your mattress is firm.
- Adopt the 'C' shape. This is also known as the 'cuddle curl' and it is a protective sleeping position. Your arm is above your baby's head to stop your pillow from encroaching near them, and your body acts as a barrier from your partner. Your legs are curled up so that your baby can't make their way down the bed either. This position also makes it less likely that you will roll.
- If you or your partner are smokers, do not co-sleep.
- If you have been drinking, taking drugs or are on any medication that could make you drowsy, do not co-sleep.
- If you are exhausted, do not co-sleep.
- It is not recommended to co-sleep if you do not exclusively breastfeed, as the risk of SIDS to bottle and combo-fed babies is higher. I personally think this is more of a grey area. We know that the risks of

SIDs reduce after 6+ months, so there may be some very responsive and sensitive parents to older babies that may feel more confident about co-sleeping. But if in doubt, don't co-sleep.

COPING WITH SLEEP CHALLENGES BABY'S HERE

Everyone around me was getting a 'sleep consultant', and miraculously, £500 later their babies were all sleeping the night through. But each time I asked them how this happened, they would give me a variation of the 'cry it out' (CIO) method, often just labelled as something else.

CIO is a method of sleep training whereby the child is put to sleep whilst they are awake and left to fall asleep on their own. There are lots of different takes on it, some are certainly less extreme and may allow you to pick up and put back down your baby, it may involve you leaving the room totally, or popping back in periodically, or staying in the room. It is typically used to try to remove a sleep association, like rocking, feeding or holding your baby to sleep, and encouraging them to 'self-soothe'. As the name implies, the child will often cry, as their usual sleep routine is drastically changed. Even sleep consultants who called themselves 'gentle' seemed to eventually get to a point in the process where they let the child cry. The idea behind self-soothing, and not needing the help of a parent to fall back to sleep, does sound really appealing, and on the face of it you think that it can only be beneficial to a baby to know how to soothe themselves. However, self-soothing is a learned developmental milestone, and it is not something that can be forced upon them. Yet, you will find that there are parents, blogs and sleep consultants out there who will show that after CIO, their babies fell asleep by themselves.

Interestingly, a study by the University of North Texas researched children who were undergoing CIO methods. Their cortisol levels, the stress hormone measured in their saliva, were found to be elevated. But all these babies eventually went to sleep. On rechecking their cortisol levels again during this apparent peaceful sleep, they were still found to be as elevated as they had been when they were actively CIO[186]. This suggests that they had not learnt to self-soothe, they probably just learnt that no one was going to help them, so they gave up and slept. That study broke my heart.

Now there is no judgement here, and you must do whatever works for you and your family. I recognise that babies cry and that you can't avoid every tear, it is how they communicate. Babies need to let it out, to know that you are not scared of their sadness, that they can be their ugliest around you, and you will still love them unconditionally. However, I also never felt comfortable letting Harris cry at night knowing that there was something I could do to ease his suffering, even if it was at the expense of my sleep and sanity – temporarily!

I remember one of my friends giving me the number of her sleep consultant, saying how her boy had gone from waking every hour to waking once a night in the space of 1 week. She reassured me that she would be as 'gentle' as you wanted. After a night of desperation, I called her. We spent 30 minutes discussing Harris' sleep patterns and what I had been doing thus far, and the answer at the end of the conversation was that I had to stop breastfeeding him to sleep and she would show me what to do instead. I told her that that wasn't on the cards, and her answer was, 'Well it sounds like the issue with his sleep is you, and when you are ready to give up feeding him to sleep, call me back.' I was livid.

I tell you this story partly because it is healthy to offload, but also as a reminder that there are many people out there selling you the dream, in this case, infant sleep. However, they do not always have your best interests at heart, and they may see a sleepless, distraught and panicked parent who has come to their wit's end and is willing to throw money at the problem, and they may take advantage. This is not to say all sleep consultants do this, on the contrary, there are plenty whose sleeping lives have been transformed with their help. But if at any point you do not feel at ease with anything they suggest, or your values do not align, walk away. You will never regret the nights that you held your crying baby, that you fed them, that you comforted them. You may, however, regret the nights that you did not. They can feel neverending at the time but they will pass soon enough. That's not to say I completely agree with the 'enjoy every moment' mantra, as a lot of moments are very hard and I'm not here for toxic positivity! But only to say that with babies and infants, everything is a stage and nothing lasts forever.

If sleep is a struggle, there are a few principles and tips you can follow to see if there is any improvement.

OPTIMISE THE BEDTIME ROUTINE

Children of most ages crave routine. At a time when everything can feel new and overwhelming for them, a steady and consistent routine can help to calm down a frayed nervous system. Consistency can also help to regulate their internal body clocks, and a predictable routine signals to your baby that it is time to wind down and prepare for sleep. Your routine can take whatever shape works for your family. For us, the bedtime routine started with rough-housing or rough-and-tumble play. This may sound counterproductive, but Harris always seemed to have excess energy just before bed, and it would never really work to put him down for sleep whilst he was jumping around. So we incorporated some time before bed to expend that energy. Depending on his age, we would either create an obstacle course of pillows to climb over, play tug of war, throw him about, crawl around with cushions on our backs that can't fall and touch the lava or roll about trying to escape the tickle monster. This gave him the sensory input he needed, let off any tension he had been building up through the day, and also allowed for some one-on-one connection time. When he was much younger and couldn't really do most of those physical things, we would make him a surprise sensory bag every night to play with instead. This didn't have to be anything special, just random things that looked and felt different – a washing sponge, bouncy ball, ribbons, garlic crusher, bubble wrap, foil – honestly, anything we could find in the house! After all of the energy was out of the way, the calming aspect of the bedtime routine would begin, we would dim the lights, have a bath, put on bedtime music, have a bit of massage, then read books. Some children will find a bath stimulating rather than relaxing, so just change things to suit your baby.

CREATE A SLEEP-INVITING ENVIRONMENT

When babies go to sleep, it is probably still early evening, and in the summer this means the sun is shining, and people are out in their gardens enjoying life and making noise. This is not particularly conducive to sleep. We invested in some blackout blinds that we could stick on the windows (foil works too), and a white-noise machine to create a soothing background noise and drown out the calamity of our neighbours imbibing in their garden. It is also worth investing in a thermostat for the bedroom. An ideal temperature for sleep is 16–18°C. It is also soporific to come from a warm environment (the bath) into a cooler environment (the room).

BE MINDFUL OF YOUR BABY'S SLEEP CUES

Recognise your baby's sleep cues so that you are not risking putting a totally awake baby to sleep who will resist, or conversely overstep the mark into the overtired zone, when your baby's screaming may prevent an easy put-down. I am often reluctant to label 'overtiredness' as a cause of not sleeping, as an overly tired baby will eventually sleep as their sleep pressure is so high. Still, they may need comforting and co-regulating to calm them down before they feel safe enough to sleep. Either way, starting the bedtime routine at the first signs of sleep cues is better for all parties involved.

DON'T BE SCARED TO TRY OUT NEW TIMINGS

If your baby's sleep schedule does not seem to work for you or them, don't be scared to switch it up. It can feel daunting to break away from the 'normal' routine, but there is no harm in trialling shorter naps, dropping naps, pushing back bedtime or waking earlier, and seeing if any of these changes help optimise your baby's sleep. Despite what many web searches try to tell you, there is no one-size-fits-all when it comes to babies' sleep schedules.

DO WHAT WORKS

You can feel like a failure when your Instagram grid is littered with photos of your friends' babies asleep so cutely in their cribs, and yours is a limpet stuck to you at all times. However, I have realised the need to work with what you've got, and, as long as you are managing, don't feel pressured to do otherwise. If you can only get your baby to sleep by breastfeeding, feed them for as long as you are happy to. If your baby only does contact naps, invest in a wrap/sling and take your baby on whatever errands you need to run whilst they sleep on you for as long as you are happy to. Or if you cannot get them to sleep in a crib at night, move the mattress to the floor (see co-sleeping, page 238) and lie next to them until they fall asleep, for as long as you are happy to.

SEEK HELP

This may come in the form of seeking support from your partner, family and friends. There is no medal for being a sleep martyr, and you are putting yourself and your baby at risk if you are exhausted, so reach out when you need it to whoever is willing to help. If it is feeds that are keeping your sleep fragmented, ask someone to take over some of the night feeds (expressed or formula), or, if this is not possible, ask someone to come early in the morning to take over whilst you get a couple of hours sleep. You should contact your GP or health visitor if you have any concerns about any red flags with your baby's sleep. As discussed above, you can also consider sleep training. Whilst helpful bedtime routines can be established earlier, some sleep training methods are not recommended until your baby is at least 4 to 6 months old. Ensure you research your sleep consultant, get recommendations from friends with similar values, use the free pre-consultation wisely to ensure you agree with their methods, and be prepared to say no to anything you feel uncomfortable with.

THIS TOO SHALL PASS

The most comforting yet annoying phrase wrapped in one. When you are going through a difficult sleep patch, you want solutions, not some wishy-washy phrase. However, there is not a truer word spoken. What seems like the apocalypse now is honestly just a phase. It will get better. Your child will start to sleep for longer. They will stop catching every cold, keeping them up. They will stop waking up for feeds. Their teeth will all come out and stop interrupting their sleep in pain. They will eventually want to sleep independently. They will do it all. Just as we did when we were growing up. So hold on to the faith that this too shall pass.

There are also several sleep myths out there that I would like to debunk so that you do not waste your time fretting over them!

Your baby should sleep through the night (STTN) by the time they are 6 months. The first issue with this is that STTN is a subjective term. One parent might define it as 6 hours, another might define it as 12 hours. The second issue is that a baby might STTN one night and not do it again for another 3 months, but does that still mean they sleep through the night? Often sleep studies adopt a binary 'ever/never' definition, so a baby who has STTN once will be defined as STTN even though they never did it again. This skews the statistics, making it seem that babies everywhere are always STTN, except for yours! Many studies are looking into this, but the statistics are so varied. Where one study suggests that 16 per cent of 6-month-olds STTN[187], another will state that only 6 per cent of 6-month-olds sleep 6 hours a night[188]. Whatever the exact number, night wakings are normal. Needing parental help to get back to sleep is normal. Most studies also agree that it's not until after 2 years that regular night waking not requiring parental attention becomes much less common. Do not let the STTN crew tell you otherwise.

Rice cereal will help them sleep better. This old-school parenting tip is often spouted out by well-meaning neighbours and relatives who say that when your baby starts to eat solids that they will wake less frequently. This may stem from the same flawed logic that breastfeeding causes broken sleep, so that if they can just eat, they won't need to wake up at night to feed anymore. Whilst there is certainly a link between the circadian rhythm, metabolism and appetite, introducing solids should be done based on your baby's developmental readiness (see weaning, page 251), not on their sleep. There is no evidence that rice cereal added to your baby's milk will improve their sleep, and if anything, you can do more harm than good by introducing a choking risk.

Breastfeeding is the cause of broken sleep. I cannot tell you the number of times I was told that if I want Harris to sleep longer stretches, I need to wean him off the breast at night. This was often followed by comments such as, 'He is just using you as a pacifier', and 'He doesn't need the feed.' Now, of course, if you want to night wean, you should be supported to do this, but do not do it because of the perceptions of others, and do not pin all your hopes on night weaning improving the night sleep (although it may for some). Your baby may not need the feed, and, quite rightly, they may be using you as a pacifier, but it is known that hunger is not the only reason your baby breastfeeds. They may be waking up for comfort and support rather than hunger, and if offering your breast is a quick and easy way of fulfilling that need, do it if you're happy to. Babies under 18 months will still need sleep support, and you will need to find another way to comfort your baby back to sleep if you choose to night wean. I don't know about you, but I would choose to fling over my breast and then fall asleep again in minutes over getting up, picking him up, rocking, bouncing or singing to sleep and then struggling to fall back to sleep again myself. I found that once Harris reached age 2, I could reason with him better and explain why I would be reducing his night feeds. I set boundaries and offered him alternative ways to settle in the night. He still woke with the same amount of frequency, but with time he was able to go back to sleep by just touching my chest. This would not have worked for him before age 2; he was just not developmentally ready. In summary, for some, night weaning may improve sleep, but there is no certainty that it will solve your sleep woes. If breastfeeding is quick, easy, reliable and you're happy to do it, crack on; you are not the cause of your child's sleep pattern. If you are struggling or it is unsustainable, for whatever reason, stop, but be prepared to step in with another form of support.

'Drowsy but awake' is the only way your child will STTN. This phrase gives me anxiety. It is the premise that when you put your child down for sleep they should not be asleep. They can be drowsy and ready to sleep but still awake. I understand where this has come from. Imagine that you are asleep in your cosy bed and have just roused from your sleep cycle; you briefly open your eyes, see that all is as it should be, and you fall back to sleep. You barely even register that you have woken. However, let's replay this situation, where you briefly open your eyes, and instead of being in your cosy bed, where you last were when you fell asleep, you are in the middle of a park. You would freak out. Then you would go back home, 'self-regulate' by trying to rationalise the situation, take some deep breaths, and eventually go back to sleep. So that being said, put your baby in this situation, they fall asleep in your arms, feeling warm, happy and protected by the only person in the world they know and trust. But when they wake up, they are on a firm, cool surface and you are not there. They, too, freak out, but they do not have the skill to self-regulate yet, so they signal for you the only way they know how, by wailing and waiting for you to de-stress and comfort them back to sleep. The theory of 'drowsy but awake' aims to annul this issue by ensuring the baby knows where they are when falling asleep and letting them fall asleep without needing any external crutches. It sounds so easy. I watched tens of videos of babies doing this, but keeping Harris awake while breastfeeding was often nigh-on impossible. This is a natural biological feature of breastfeeding. Your breast milk is full of wonderful hormones whose specific drive is to get your baby to sleep, so we would skip the drowsy stage and go straight to sleep. Or if by some miracle I managed to keep Harris awake, he would scream as soon as he was being lowered into the crib. It was so counterproductive, as the act of screaming just woke him up even more. It didn't matter how I did it – swaddled, unswaddled, sideways, bum first – he screamed, adding to the feeling of failure. Eventually, I gave up, realising that the kind of babies that are happy to be put down drowsy but awake, are probably also the kind of babies that are 'better' sleepers. Interestingly, a large study found no statistically significant difference between the sleep of babies who were put to sleep awake against those who fell asleep breastfeeding or in arms[189]. So 'drowsy but awake' can enter the rubbish bin pile, and you can regain your sanity.

I cannot pretend to be a sleep expert. I did not, and still don't, three years on, have a child who 'sleeps through the night', so I am not the poster girl for sleep. But at least I am honest about it, and I can tell you that nothing prepares you for how much your baby will need you, day and night. We don't all have that village that is supposedly coming to our rescue, we still have to get up and go to work, and none of this is convenient on fragmented sleep.

I struggled massively with coming to terms with Harris' sleep initially; I panic-bought books, scoured the internet and followed every sleep expert on social media. The only thing that really helped was realising that sleep is a biological function that is out of our conscious control. There is not necessarily a solution to sleep, and there isn't an exact formula or process you have to follow. I needed to understand that my baby would just have to reach his sleep milestone in his own sweet time. Finding ways around the broken sleep became my saviour.

Feeding to sleep might not work for you, co-sleeping might scare you, floor beds might ruin the aesthetics of your house, and wearing your baby may not be your thing, but these were all the techniques that meant I could get on with my day and night, and not resent my baby or have a total meltdown. I forgave myself for not being the mother that other people seemed to be, and I let go of the fear and anxiety that I was holding onto around sleep.

Harris now, at three, sleeps in his own bed for the beginning of the night, and when he wakes in the middle of the night, he comes to sleep in bed with us. This might not look like the picture I imagined in my head when I first found out I was pregnant and planned the perfect nursery, but it works for us. I get to wake up every morning with my son's angelic face sleeping next to me (and often his foot in my face), and, truthfully, I wouldn't have it any other way. One day he will wake in the night and not want to sleep with us anymore, and that day will be bittersweet.

SLEEP: A TIRED MAMMA'S SUMMARY

Importance of sleep: sleep is crucial for physical growth, brain development, skill consolidation and memory organisation. Sleep allows the release of growth hormones, supports immune system optimisation and aids tissue repair. Well-rested infants exhibit improved focus, alertness, stable moods and reduced irritability, better equipping them to face daily challenges.

Newborn sleep patterns: while sleep charts provide guidance, not all babies conform to these averages. Watch out for red flags that might indicate underlying sleep issues, such as excessive daytime sleepiness, irregular breathing, distress, developmental concerns or restless sleep. While these flags may not necessarily indicate problems, seeking healthcare advice is recommended. Potential health conditions affecting sleep include gastroesophageal reflux disease (GERD), respiratory conditions, pain, neurological conditions and iron deficiency.

Sleep cycles: consist of non-rapid eye movement (NREM) and rapid eye movement (REM) sleep stages, crucial for brain development. Newborns often require assistance to transition between sleep cycles. Wake windows, the time between sleeps, play a role in falling asleep and achieving restful sleep. While wake windows can be helpful, each baby has unique sleep patterns, and relying solely on prescribed wake windows may not suit all infants.

Sleep progression: there are a number of stages when sleep can become a challenge. This is usually due to developmental leaps in your baby.

Newborn sleep progression: challenges during this phase include immature circadian rhythms, frequent nappy changes, comfort needs and night feeds. Regulating circadian rhythms becomes essential.

Four-month sleep progression: as babies become more alert and responsive, sleep cycles lengthen. Establishing a bedtime routine helps introduce sleep cues.

Six-month sleep progression: increased brain activity due to motor skill development can lead to restlessness. Introducing solids and maintaining daytime stimulation helps manage night wakings.

Eight–ten-month sleep progression: crawling and separation anxiety can affect sleep. Creating a sense of security through games and maintaining a consistent bedtime routine is crucial.

Twelve-month sleep progression: walking and increased brain activity may lead to more active sleep. Encouraging outdoor exploration and providing comfort and support can help manage sleep changes.

Sudden Infant Death Syndrome (SIDS): the sudden and unexplained death of an infant under one. There are a number of risk factors for this.

Intrinsic risk factors for SIDS: factors like male sex, prematurity, low birth weight, genetic polymorphisms and prenatal exposure to drugs can increase vulnerability.

Extrinsic risk factors SIDS: unsafe sleep positions, sharing sleep surfaces, overheating, soft bedding and inappropriate sleep surfaces contribute to SIDS risk.

Recommendations to reduce SIDS risk: include back sleeping, room-sharing, avoiding smoking and alcohol, breastfeeding and using pacifiers.

COPING WITH SLEEP CHALLENGES

Optimising bedtime routine: consistent routines and sensory activities before bed help regulate sleep.

Creating a sleep-inviting environment: blackout blinds, white noise and suitable room temperature contribute to better sleep.

Recognising sleep cues: identifying cues helps prevent overtiredness and supports better sleep.

Trying new timings: flexibility in sleep schedules can improve sleep quality.

Getting support: reaching out for help from family, friends and professionals is encouraged.

CHAPTER 9

WEANING BABY'S HERE

Weaning is the process of gradually introducing solid foods to your baby. You will be transitioning your baby from an exclusive diet of breast or formula feeding to one including solids and other liquids. Parents are often really excited to start the weaning process and see their baby's face when they try a brand-new taste or texture. It is exciting, but it also marks the end of an easy life (feeding-wise)! Whilst they only drank milk, it was either on tap (breast) or a quick mix and a shake (formula) away. Once they start weaning, your preparation levels have to go up a notch and your cleaning products have to be on standby. This was a welcome thing for me whilst I was still on maternity leave. Maybe it is not acceptable to admit, but I was so bored of the same routine, I longed for another project, and I made baby-led weaning it.

WHY DO WE WEAN?

We often talk about how perfectly formulated breast milk is, and formula milk has been made to mimic this. So, if milk is so encompassing, why would we wean? This is because as babies grow, their nutritional needs change. What was a perfect recipe for a newborn is no longer able to provide the nutrients that a growing baby needs. The iron requirement is an example of this. When your baby is born they are supplied with iron from your placenta, but these iron stores begin to deplete and, unfortunately, breast milk provides little iron. Solid foods that are rich in iron, like meat, lentils and fortified foods, can help meet this iron requirement.

As well as the nutritional needs of your baby changing, so too does their curiosity. They have seen you eating every day, and as they become older, they too will want to explore this magical thing that you keep putting in your mouth. Weaning will help to satisfy this curiosity of tastes and textures, as well as help to support their oral and motor skills and coordination. It can also help support social interactions and promote a sense of inclusion by allowing them to participate in family meals. Being exposed to a wide variety of flavours, textures and food groups may also broaden their taste preferences and promote a varied and balanced diet later in life.

There is some evidence that weaning also protects us from allergies. Many parents are scared about giving their baby a common allergen food, like nuts, for example. However, data suggests that introducing peanut products into babies' diets by 6 months could reduce the risk of peanut allergy by 77 per cent[190]. (This goes without saying, but please don't start giving babies whole nuts! There are many resources available to teach you how to safely prepare different foods for different ages.)

HOW DO I KNOW WHEN MY BABY IS READY TO WEAN?

Most babies start showing signs of readiness for solid foods around the age of 6 months, though some may be ready earlier and others later. It is important to look for these signs before starting the weaning process. Some studies suggest that starting earlier than 4 months, or before they are ready can lead to an increased risk of chronic disease, obesity, coeliac disease, as well as poor nutrition outcomes because of displacement of nutrient-rich milk. There is also evidence that suggests it can increase the risk of gastrointestinal infections, resulting in diarrhoea and/or vomiting[191]. Furthermore, if your baby is breastfed, exclusively breast-feeding also decreases the risks of other infections including ear and respiratory tract infections, so curtailing this too early may result in these infections becoming more prevalent[192].

If you can answer yes to all of these questions, and your baby is above 4 months old, you can consider starting the weaning process:

- Are they sitting up unaided, with their head held steady?
- Are they able to swallow food? Babies have a tongue thrust reflex which makes their tongue stick out when something is touched to their lips or tongue. It is there to protect them from choking on food or foreign objects. It gradually starts to fade between 4 and 6 months. Whilst it might not be totally gone when you start weaning, it needs to be diminished enough that they can actually swallow.
- Can they reach for and hold food, and be coordinated enough to put it in their mouths?

Please note that chewing their fists, wanting more milk and waking up more than usual at night are not signs that they need to wean.

HOW TO PREPARE FOR WEANING

It's hard not to get carried away buying bamboo plates in the shape of an elephant when you get started, but there are several items you can prepare yourself with that can make the process more enjoyable for all parties and go more smoothly:

Highchair – these come in such a variety of budgets, styles and sizes that it can be overwhelming to decide which to buy. However, there are a number of factors to consider that will help your baby eat.

Body support – the highchair needs to be supportive enough so that the baby can sit comfortably upright without slipping down. This might require buying additional padded cushions. They should also be sitting with a 90-degree angle at the hips and knees so they are not leaning forwards or backwards.

Foot rest – make sure there is a footrest to allow your baby better stability when sitting, preferably an adjustable one to accommodate your baby's growth.

Close to the table – this is already a feature if you choose a highchair with a tray. However, if you choose one that you place at a table, ensure the chair can fit close enough to the table that your baby does not have to make a significant reach to get to the food, and it allows them to rest their elbows on the table.

Cup – whilst their primary fluid intake will still be breast or formula milk, you can offer sips of water. It might be messy, but it's best to use an open or free-flow cup without a valve, as they help your baby learn to sip and are best for your baby's teeth.

Bowl – the main prerequisites are that the bowl/plate is indestructible and easy to clean. Suction weaning sets are also useful to avoid the plate being flung across the room. However, they do not stick on all surfaces, so check that your highchair tray or dining room table is suction-compatible before investing in them. If you want to be able to put different foods in different segments, you can also consider plates that are sectioned.

Utensils – if you followed baby-led weaning for the early days, I would just let your baby explore the food with their hands. Most babies are happy to do this for a while as it introduces them to textures and helps them develop their grip and hand–eye coordination. If you want to start them off early, or they start becoming interested in using your utensils, then you can get them a set of their own to become accustomed to. They don't need any special utensils, but it can make it easier for them if they are the right size, and have an ergonomic grip to make it easy for them to use. It is also safer if they are chowing down on a soft spoon or fork rather than a metal one, so perhaps consider plastic or silicone initially. I bought a few different sets, all of differing shapes, colours and sizes, and let Harris choose which he wanted to use. He definitely built a preference for one set, which I think felt better in his hands, so it can be a trial-and-error process.

Ice cube tray – you can buy specific freezer trays for weaning, but I found ice cube trays worked just as well. They are just very handy for batch cooking and then freezing, in baby-size portions to use over the coming weeks or months, as something easy and homemade to grab when your baby is hungry! Just check that your ice cube trays are BPA (Bisphenol-A) free to ensure they are food safe.

Bib – weaning is a messy business, and if you want any of those beautiful clothes that you were gifted at the baby shower to remain so, a bib is needed. Bibs can come in coverall style, or the type that has a scoop or pocket to catch the food. Harris was pretty reluctant to wear bibs, so he ate in just a nappy a lot of the time!

Messy mat – these are just large wipe-clean mats that you can put under your baby's highchair, so at the end of the meal you just scoop the whole thing up, shake it into your bin and wipe it clean. It will save time and your lovely flooring. They can also be used for arts and crafts, so they have longevity.

Blender – if you are planning parent-led weaning, a blender is useful to make the purées. Even with baby-led weaning, they can be helpful to have to make your baby falafels or the like. There are specific blenders and steamers that you can buy for baby weaning, and whilst I am sure they can be useful, they are not entirely necessary. My usual blender sufficed for us.

Patience – as with most things in the baby world, some babies take to weaning quickly with little fuss, and others seem disinterested and it feels like they reject everything. Patience is key, and even if they do not seem to like something, keep offering it; it can take over ten tries before your baby becomes used to the texture or taste.

Baby-led weaning versus parent-led

Baby-led weaning (BLW) is an approach that allows babies to feed themselves with appropriately sized, soft and easily graspable pieces of food that they can hold and bring to their mouths on their own. This can encourage independence, giving them a sense of autonomy in choosing what they want to eat and how much of it. It will also promote self-feeding skills, developing their fine motor skills, hand–eye coordination and chewing skills. It allows them to explore and understand the different tastes, colours and textures of food, which may help them develop a broader range of tastes and preferences. With simple and minor adaptations, it can also allow the baby to join in on family meals, adding to feelings of inclusion and social interaction and allowing you to model healthy eating habits.

However, BLW is undoubtedly messy, as half of that avocado will be smeared in their hair within 3 minutes of mealtime. It can also mean that some babies get off to a slightly slower start with weaning as they develop the skills required for self-feeding. Whilst this is unlikely to affect them initially, if it is prolonged, or there are certain foods the baby refuses to try, there is a potential risk of an inadequate nutrient intake. The most common concern of parents with BLW is the choking risk. Although the aim is to negate the risk as much as possible by offering appropriate foods (see below), there may be a higher risk of choking when self-feeding. I recommend all parents undertake a paediatric first aid course (often included in antenatal classes) to educate themselves on what to do if your baby chokes. There are lots of BLW books out there to get some great recipe ideas from. I used the book *Young Gums* by Beth Bentley. Whilst it is not an exclusive BLW book, it had loads of inspiration for BLW meals and the food was genuinely tasty, so it meant that we were all able to eat the same foods as family, which was important to me. As time went by and I felt more confident with the weaning process, I just learnt to adapt our usual recipes to be baby-safe.

Parent-led weaning (PLW), on the other hand, involves the baby being spoon-fed purée. This allows the parent to have more control over what the baby eats, ensuring each spoonful is balanced and nutritionally dense. Although it may take more preparation time to steam and blend, it can often save time on how long the meal takes to eat and on the cleaning after. A key advantage is the reduced risk of choking as you can mash or blend the purée into an appropriate texture that is easier for your baby to eat. The downsides of PLW include not promoting self-feeding skills, and less independence. As they are not exposed to a wide variety of textures and tastes early on, it may impact on food acceptance and tolerance. Finally, PLW may not fully integrate the baby into family meals, which can mean they miss out on that social interaction.

There is no right or wrong method, and these two approaches do not need to be mutually exclusive. Many parents will choose a combination of both best to fit their needs and their baby's needs.

WHAT FOODS TO START WITH

It seems an incredibly boring start to what can be an enjoyable journey. However, it is best to begin with single-ingredient foods. So put those baby cookbooks away initially, and focus on one food at a time, waiting a few days before introducing another. This helps you identify any allergies or sensitivities.

Anything can cause an allergy, but there are some more common culprits. It is still important to offer these foods when you start weaning, just in small amounts and one at a time. These include, though are not limited to:

- Cow's milk
- Eggs
- Gluten (wheat, barley and rye)
- Nuts
- Seeds
- Soya
- Shellfish
- Fish

I recommend that you only introduce a new food when your child is well, so that you can ensure any symptoms are related to the food and not an underlying illness. It is also wise to introduce the new food early in the day so that you have several hours to observe your baby and see if any symptoms manifest.

It is tempting just to give your baby crowd-pleasers like fruit or sweet vegetables to start with, as you know you are more likely to get a positive response, but it is advisable to offer the more savoury foods initially to get them used to different flavours. This may help develop their palates and help to prevent fussy eating.

If you are going down the BLW route, prepare baby-sized batons. At 6 months old, your baby will use their whole hand to pick things up as they have not developed their pincer grip yet. This means that the food needs to be narrow enough for them to close their hand around. It also needs to be long enough so that the food will actually stick out above their gripped fist. The food must be soft enough to squish between your fingers, but not too soft that it disintegrates in their grip. Examples of some healthy BLW options to start with include:

- Steamed broccoli
- Steamed asparagus
- Cucumber strips
- Avocado strips (if they were too slippery, I rolled them in oats to help Harris grip, or I would leave the lower half of the skin on)
- Steamed or roasted root vegetables (carrots, parsnips, butternut squash)
- Steamed baby sweetcorn
- Cheese strips
- Quartered hard-boiled egg or strips of omelette

Once your baby has gone through a fair number of single-ingredient foods, you can start to become more adventurous, and even cook the same meals as the rest of the family, being mindful to limit additions of salt and sugar.

It is helpful to introduce meat to your baby as it is high in iron, the stores of which start to deplete from 6 months onwards. It can be offered as a purée when PLW, but in BLW it is best to either use ground meat formed into a meatball (or more easily held, meatlog!) or into strips of soft-cooked meat that your baby is most likely to suck and gnaw on. They can still absorb some of the nutrients this way, so don't worry if their little gummy mouths aren't actually able to eat it. For those that do not eat meat or fish, there are other sources of iron. This includes fortified breakfast cereals, green leafy vegetables like spinach, kale and cabbage, and beans, lentils and chickpeas. It is harder for our bodies to absorb iron in its vegetarian form, so larger quantities are often needed. However, there are ways to help increase this absorption, including eating it alongside foods high in vitamin C, so consider adding foods like strawberries or citrus fruit to their iron-rich meal.

In terms of fluids, just offer sips of water to your baby. If they are under 6 months, this should be cooled-down boiled water. After 6 months, it can be straight from the tap. I tend to avoid bottled mineral water, as it has a higher salt content, which is unhealthy for your baby.

FOOD NO-NOS

We want to provide a diverse, healthy and well-balanced diet. However, there are some foods that should be off the menu or limited:

Salt – your baby's kidneys are not mature enough to be able to process high amounts of salt. They don't know yet how salt can enhance flavour, so they do not know what they are missing yet, so steer clear of adding salt to any of their food, and be mindful of the salt content of any shop-bought foods. Babies under a year should have less than 1g of salt per day, less than 0.4g of sodium per day.

Sugar – added sugar contributes to tooth decay and unhealthy eating habits, so avoid adding sugar to anything for as long as they can remain ignorant about it! Grandparents will consistently want to give them 'a little treat', but try to reinforce the concept that sugary foods are not recommended in babies under 1 year.

Raw shellfish – this carries a risk of food poisoning and should be avoided in babies.

Runny eggs – if the eggs have the red 'British Lion stamp' printed on them, it is safe for them to eat runny, but if they do not they need to be fully cooked.

Shark/swordfish/marlin – these fish have higher levels of mercury and can affect your baby's nervous system.

Honey – this can contain spores of bacteria that cause botulism, which is a rare but serious condition caused by the toxins made by the bacteria *Clostridium botulinum*. The toxins can attack the nervous system and result in paralysis. The paralysis is usually temporary, but if they affect the muscles that control breathing it can be fatal. The spores found in honey are harmless in older children and adults, but it is recommended that honey is avoided until your baby is at least 1 year old.

Cow milk as a primary drink – until your baby is 1, cow's milk should not be given as a primary drink. Breast milk or formula should be their main source of nutrition. You can use whole milk in cooking for your baby from 6 months onwards.

Choking hazards – whole nuts, seeds and popcorn are all considered choking hazards. Nuts and seeds are very nutritious but should be offered in other forms like nut/seed butter or finely ground. Spread the nut/seed butter thinly on bread rather than offering it in a lump or on a spoon, which can still be a choking hazard. A little tip I picked up was that if your nut butter was too clumpy, you could heat it in the microwave until it was warm, which helped to smooth it out to spread it thinner.

Hard fruit and vegetables – these must be cooked to soften. Although grapes and blueberries are soft due to their shape they are also considered a choking hazard and should be quartered (grapes) or squashed flat (blueberries).

Ultra-processed foods – where possible, minimise highly processed foods, as they offer little nutritional value and contain lots of additional ingredients that are at best useless and at worst harmful. Look at the labels, and if there are ingredients in there that you wouldn't recognise as staples in a kitchen, avoid them.

Low-fat foods – fat gives babies energy and provides some vitamins that are only found in fat, so choose full-fat dairy foods to offer the highest nutrient content in the smallest amount of food.

Juice – although juices seem like an easy-to-attain source of vitamins, they also contain sugars and are acidic, which means they can cause tooth decay. Ideally, you should only offer your child sips of water, but if you do choose to offer juice, always dilute it well with water and offer it in a feeding cup at mealtimes only.

Do not wean before 4 months – no matter how developed you think your baby is, it is unsafe to wean them any earlier than this.

READY-PREPARED BABY FOOD

We would all love to be perfect mothers, preparing everything from scratch and feeding our babies the god's nectar. However, life is rarely that kind to us, and it is normal and acceptable that you may need to buy ready-prepared food for your baby at times. Although they are more expensive than homemade food, they are undoubtedly convenient, particularly handy when travelling and don't have access to a kitchen, or when you are back at work and evenings become even more rushed than usual!

It is more important what you are feeding your baby than what packaging it comes in, so ideally choose foods specifically made for babies. They are often more 'natural' and try to keep ingredients and added preservatives to a minimum; they are also less likely to contain added salt or sugar. Whilst many of the baby food pouches are marketed as savoury, have a look at their ingredients, as I often find that they contain a lot of fruit too, probably to make it more palatable to babies. Avoid ready-prepared baby food with ingredients that you don't recognise as actual foods. Furthermore, it is not recommended to let your baby suck the food out of the pouches, as this may contribute to tooth decay. Instead, squeeze the contents out into little spoons for them.

WHAT DOES AN ALLERGIC REACTION LOOK LIKE?

Around 5 per cent of 0–2-year-olds have a diagnosed food allergy[193]. The most common allergens in babies are cow's milk, egg, peanut, soya, wheat and fish. As you will be introducing foods into your baby's diet one by one, it will help you identify if one of these is an allergen. There are two main types of food allergies, Immunoglobulin E (IgE) mediated and non-IgE mediated.

IgE-mediated food allergies trigger an immediate reaction in response to the allergenic food. The IgE antibodies recognise the specific allergen and activate mast cells and basophils, releasing histamines and other inflammatory mediators. The reaction is usually within minutes to a couple of hours (most commonly within 30 minutes) and can range from mild reactions like hives and itching to severe reactions like anaphylaxis. Though to reassure you, anaphylaxis in children under 12 months is rare. Once the allergen is removed from the body, the reaction tends to resolve quickly too. The most common IgE-mediated food allergy in babies is egg. These allergies are often diagnosed through skin prick tests, blood tests (to measure specific IgE levels) and food challenges under medical supervision.

IgE does not drive non-IgE mediated food allergies but instead by other immune system components, like T cells, which are involved in the inflammatory response to the food allergen. The reaction tends to be delayed, taking hours to days to manifest. Often with symptoms like diarrhoea, vomiting and eczema. The symptoms can also persist for longer. The most common non-IgE food allergy in babies is cow's milk. It can be more challenging to diagnose non-IgE mediated food allergies and usually involves keeping a food diary, trialling elimination diets and food challenges.

Not all reactions to food are because of allergies. For example, certain foods like tomatoes, strawberries and citrus fruits can irritate the skin around the mouth, making it red and sore. You do not need to avoid this food, rather just apply a barrier, like a moisturiser, around the mouth before your baby eats these foods to reduce the contact reaction.

	IgE mediated food allergy	Non-IgE mediated food allergy
Duration	Rapid onset	Delayed onset
Symptoms	Hives Itching Coughing Wheezing Acute vomiting Swelling of lips, tongue or face Anaphylaxis	Vomiting Diarrhoea Stomach pain Bloating Reflux Eczema

As you saw, milk is on the list of allergens. This is something we offer to our babies from the moment they are born. Formula milk in the UK is based on modified cow's milk. Cow's Milk Protein Allergy (CMPA) is more likely to occur in formula-fed babies, but if your baby has been drinking formula milk without any issues, the risk of them developing an allergy to cow's milk when weaning is low.

Whilst CMA in babies who are exclusively breastfed is low (<1 in 100), they are at greater risk of developing this allergy when it is introduced into the diet on weaning[194]. Babies who show signs of milk allergy when breastfeeding should continue to breastfeed, but the mother may need to eliminate cow's milk from her diet.

If your baby exhibits signs of an allergic reaction, your action will depend on its severity.

Mild or moderate reaction

- Symptoms – runny or blocked nose, itchy or watery eyes, sneezing, coughing, itchy rash.
- Remove the food that you think is the allergen.
- If they are under 1 year old, speak to your GP/111 regarding antihistamines, as in under ones they are prescription-only medication. If they are over 1 year old, you can give them antihistamines from the pharmacy.
- If you are unsure that it is just mild, call 999.
- Don't offer that food again until you have sought medical advice.

Severe reaction

- Symptoms – persistent cough, swollen tongue, hoarse voice, difficulty swallowing, noisy breathing/wheezing, pale, floppy, sleepy, unconscious.
- Lay them down (if they are struggling to breathe, you can prop them up).
- Elevate their legs.
- If they have a prescribed autoinjector pen, use it.
- Call 999.
- Start CPR if unresponsive and not breathing.
- If there's no improvement after 5 minutes, use the autoinjector pen again.

ALLERGY-PRONE BABIES

Weaning can feel more challenging when you have a baby who is at risk of developing an allergy, like babies with eczema, and existing food allergies like CMA. Up until recently in the UK, these allergy prone babies were advised to avoid peanuts until around 3 years of age, however, two major studies have led to this advice being totally flipped on its head.

The Learning Early About Peanut Allergy (LEAP) study[195] and the EAT Study[196] both looked into the early introduction of allergens in babies. Off the back of these studies, the recommendation is that babies with a known risk factor for food allergy should introduce cooked egg and then peanut alongside other solids from 4 months of age, if they are developmentally ready. When introducing peanuts into your baby's diet, make sure your baby is well and any eczema is well-controlled, and choose a day when you are at home and you have time to observe your baby for at least 2 hours after they have eaten the food containing peanuts. The peanuts would need to be prepared in a safe baby-friendly way and you will need to start with a very small amount (as small as a grain of rice) of peanut butter initially and then gradually increase the amount on a daily basis. Usually this is offered as a thinned, smooth peanut butter, prepared by adding it to a few teaspoons of cooled boiled water, which can then be given to your baby as is, or mixed with a suitable baby cereal or other wet foods. Alternatively, it could be puréed with fruit, vegetables or baby cereal.

Introducing peanuts would be with the support of a specialist and they will give you an individualised regime of how to prepare it, how much peanut butter to give and how and when to increase the dose. If the baby does not have these risk factors, we should continue to only introduce these allergens at around 6 months of age. The studies found that by actively trying to exclude or delay the introduction of allergens, we may be increasing the risk of developing an allergy to that food.

CHOKING VERSUS GAGGING

Whilst both of these physiological responses can occur when introducing your baby to solids, and they both do look alarming to parents, there are significant differences.

Gagging is actually a protective reflex, to prevent the baby from choking. It is a normal and essential reflex that occurs when something touches the back of the throat or triggers the soft palate. The baby will make a retching or coughing sound that helps push the food to the front of their mouth. It is not harmful and as the baby learns to manage solid foods, this will become less frequent.

Conversely, choking is potentially life threatening. It occurs when the food becomes stuck in the throat or windpipe, obstructing the flow of air. Signs of choking can include difficulty breathing, inability to cry or make sounds, and a blue tint to the lips and skin. Unlike with gagging, which you can allow your baby to manipulate the food back out, choking requires immediate action. It is important to know the difference between the two, because performing some of the following actions if your baby is simply gagging can actually push the food further in and cause choking. Although it can feel triggering, I recommend familiarising yourself with how the two actions differ by watching them online on places like YouTube.

What to do if your baby is choking:

1. Give up to five back blows – hold the baby facing down along your forearm and thigh, support their head and neck but ensure their head is lower than their bottom. Hit them firmly with the heel of your hand on their back between their shoulder blades, up to five times.
2. Turn them over and pick out any obvious obstruction, but do not do a blind sweep of the mouth as this risks pushing it further down the throat.
3. Give up to five chest thrusts – with your baby lying facing upwards along your thighs, and their head and neck supported, place two fingers in the middle of their chest just below the nipple line. Push down sharply five times.
4. Call 999 and repeat the five back blows and five chest thrusts until the ambulance arrives.
5. If at any point the baby becomes unresponsive, start CPR.

The above instructions should merely be an aide-memoire and should not replace attending a paediatric first aid course.

VITAMIN SUPPLEMENTATION

In the first 6 months, babies generally get all their nutrition to support growth and development from breast milk or formula milk, and then when they start weaning, their diverse diet will contribute to filling any nutrient gaps. This is with the exception of vitamin D in breastfed babies.

Breastfed babies do need to take daily vitamin D supplements from birth. Vitamin D is needed for bone health, and has also been implicated in immune health. Breast milk contains some vitamin D, but it may not be in a sufficient amount, especially if the mother is insufficient or deficient in vitamin D. Providing they are drinking more than 500ml a day, formula-fed babies do not need to take additional vitamin D as the formula is already fortified with it. The dose of vitamin D up to the age of 1 is 8.5 to 10 micrograms of vitamin D. The dose for children aged 1 to 4 years old is 10 micrograms.

To further supplement the nutritional requirements of a weaning baby, the UK government recommends that children aged 6 months to 5 years take daily supplements containing vitamins A, C and D[197]. If they are still consuming more than 500ml of formula a day, they do not need to be given these additional supplements as formula is already fortified with these. You can buy vitamin drop supplements which contain all three of these vitamins combined. Just ensure that you are not giving additional vitamin D if it is already in the combined supplement.

There are many different vitamin drops on the market. I would look at the following when assessing them.

- Do they contain vitamins A, C and D?
- Do they meet the recommended doses for your baby's age group?
- Do they have added sugars or sweeteners in them?
- Do they have any additional nutrients in them?

WEANING: A TIRED MAMMA'S SUMMARY

Signs of readiness for weaning: include a baby sitting up unaided, ability to swallow food and coordination to reach for and hold food. It's important to wait until a baby is around 4–6 months old before introducing solids.

Baby-led weaning (BLW): involves letting babies feed themselves with appropriately sized soft foods, promoting independence and self-feeding skills.

Parent-led weaning (PLW): involves spoon-feeding purées, allowing parents more control over the baby's diet.

Foods to avoid: include high-salt and high-sugar foods, raw shellfish, runny eggs without the British Lion stamp, certain fish due to mercury content, honey and choking hazards like whole nuts and popcorn.

Allergies: around 5 per cent of infants aged from birth to 2 years old have diagnosed food allergies, with common allergens including cow's milk, egg, peanut, soya, wheat and fish. Two main types of food allergies are Immunoglobulin E (IgE) mediated and non-IgE mediated. IgE mediated allergies trigger immediate reactions, while non-IgE mediated allergies tend to manifest with delayed symptoms. Symptoms of allergies include hives, itching, coughing, wheezing, vomiting, diarrhoea and eczema.

Allergy-prone babies: recent studies suggest introducing allergenic foods early to reduce the risk of allergies. This includes babies with eczema and existing allergies.

Gagging and choking during weaning: gagging is a protective reflex, while choking is a potentially life-threatening situation. Learn, before you start weaning, what to do if your baby is choking.

CHAPTER 10

TEETHING BABY'S HERE

The arrival of those tiny white Tic-Tacs in your baby's gums are utterly adorable. It transforms their geriatric gummy smiles into the classic Pampers advert baby. It also signals the milestone of them being more able to chomp on different foods and textures. However, this milestone is not always an easy one for you or your baby, and can be met with sleepless nights. But there are ways to soothe your baby and make this pearly white transition easier.

WHAT IS TEETHING?

Teething is the process of your baby's primary teeth erupting through the gums. These teeth are sometimes referred to as their milk teeth or baby teeth. This usually starts from around 6 months, but it can be as early as 3 months or as late as 1 year. In some cases, babies are even born with teeth. Most children will have their complete set of primary teeth by the age of 2 to 3 years old. Although these time-frames can vary with children, a guideline for the order of which your baby's teeth will appear is as follows:

Age	Tooth	Location
5–7 months	Bottom incisors	Bottom front teeth
6–8 months	Upper incisors	Top front teeth

Age	Tooth	Location
9–11 months	Top lateral incisors	Either side of top front teeth
10–12 months	Bottom lateral incisors	Either side of bottom front teeth
12–16 months	First molars	Back teeth
16–20 months	Canines	Between the lateral incisors and first molars
20–30 months	Second molars	Behind the first molars

SIGNS AND SYMPTOMS OF TEETHING

Some babies sail through teething with barely a whimper, other babies really suffer. One of the first signs of teething can be an increase in drooling, with your baby's chin and chest covered in saliva. They often try to find relief by gnawing on anything they can get their hands on, including toys, books and their own hands. You may observe them pulling at their ears or rubbing at their cheeks as the pain can radiate to these areas, and you may see that one cheek is more flushed. The pain may also make them more irritable and fussy, disrupting their sleep and their appetite. When you look in their mouths, the gums around the erupting tooth may appear red and swollen, and you might notice they flinch, cry or pull back if you touch it due to the tenderness. Some babies develop a mild temperature (<38 degrees), but do be mindful to ensure there is no other potential cause of the fever before dismissing it as teething. Despite popular belief, no evidence suggests that teething causes diarrhoea.

HOW TO HELP YOUR BABY

As you can see from the above teething schedule, it can be a gruelling and intense 3 years of regular teething, so you will want to do everything you can to limit the pain and disruption it can cause.

Gum massage – gently massage your baby's gum with a clean finger. The pressure may offer some relief.

Teething toys/rings – teething toys and rings give your baby something safe to gnaw on. Many of them also allow you to chill them in the fridge to soothe their gums further. Don't place them in the freezer as the extreme cold can damage your baby's gums.

Food – if your baby is already weaning and developmentally ready, you can either offer cool and soft foods like melon or chilled applesauce, or you can offer foods that they can chew on, like vegetable sticks or crusty bread. There are plenty of teething rusks/biscuits that you can buy, too, but check they do not have any added sugar in them.

Drool protection – as they are likely to be drooling more, and the saliva can roll down the chin, neck and chest, regularly wipe them to prevent a rash. You can also use a physical barrier like a bib for the neck and chest and a moisturiser barrier around the mouth.

Pain relief – if your baby is in pain with teething, you can consider pain relief like paracetamol and ibuprofen if they are over 3 months.

Love – lots of extra love, cuddles and distraction can go a long way to comfort your baby.

Teething gels – there are various teething gels available, some that are cooling and soothing, others that have anaesthetic to numb the area. As there is a lack of evidence for their effectiveness, it is recommended that you try the above non-medical options first.

HOW TO CARE FOR YOUR BABY'S TEETH

As soon as that first tooth pops out, you can start the toothbrushing fiasco! In my experience as a mum, babies (and toddlers) don't like toothbrushing, though I hear through the parental grapevine that this isn't the case for everyone. For our family it was always met with a lot of resistance, but it is also non-negotiable, and you need to brush their teeth twice daily to ensure their oral health.

You may not think that milk teeth are that important as they are only temporary, however, they do have a significant role in the alignment and spacing of their permanent teeth, as well as for the development of their speech and eating. So taking care of these placeholder teeth is necessary.

BRUSHING TEETH

Purchase age-appropriate toothpaste, as they have different amounts of fluoride in them. Similarly, an age-appropriate toothbrush is also required for the size of the head and softness of the bristles. At the beginning, we used the silicone finger toothbrush for Harris, which allowed me to control the brushing in such a wriggly little one. But as he got used to brushing and he observed our toothbrushes, he was more interested in using a 'proper' toothbrush.

Up until the age of 3, you only need to use a smear of toothpaste, so that tube lasts a while. However, you tend to go through the toothbrushes quite quickly, as babies can't help but bite them. We were replacing Harris' toothbrush every 2 or 3 months.

You might find that sitting your baby on your lap with their head against your chest gives you the best angle to brush their teeth. Brush in small circles for at least 2 minutes (if they only have one tooth, I think we can safely say you do not need to do it for this long. Just do what you can!), attempting to brush all surfaces, then encourage them to spit. You do not need to rinse the mouth.

Do this twice daily, one of these times needs to be before bed, and the other can be at any time that works for you, though I find that getting them into the habit of brushing in the morning is helpful when you then need to start getting them ready for nursery, as it settles the routine.

TRICKS

If, like me, you have a child that battles tooth brushing time, there are some tips that you might find helpful.

What's your flavour? – it turns out Harris hated mint. We had been using mild mint toothpaste and thought we would try a different flavour to see if he was any more receptive, and it was a gamechanger. Apparently, he's more of a bubblegum or Tutti Frutti man!

Give them control – when they feel so out of control of a situation and, as with much of their infant lives, are having things done to them with no consent, it can help to give them control over something. We bought Harris a few different-coloured toothbrushes and let him choose which one we used each day. I can't say if it made a huge difference to our toothbrushing experience, but it was a harmless way of making him feel like he had a choice.

Distraction – this is a tool used for everything in parenthood. When Harris was distracted with something else, he wouldn't notice the toothbrushing as much. We started brushing his teeth while in the bath to distract him with water play.

Sing a song – you can make up a toothbrushing song to make it more fun. Or if you are devoid of musical talent like me, I just used the 'Hey Duggee' toothbrushing song, which lasts exactly 2 minutes, the amount of time you should brush for.

Copycat – kids love to copy what you do. So it may help to brush your teeth simultaneously as they brush so that they feel part of the crew. We even got to the point where Harris would brush my teeth (I ended up gagging a lot!) as I brushed his.

Let them brush their teeth – it will be an entirely ineffective brush, but they will feel like they are achieving big things. Just ensure that you supervise them properly, and after they have had a go, you can do it 'properly'.

DENTIST

You can book their first dentist appointment when that first tooth comes through. There won't be much of an examination at this point, and it will probably just involve a quick mouth open, mouth shut. Still, it is important to get your baby used to going to the dentist regularly (usually 6-monthly, though the dentist might suggest a different schedule for you). The dentist will also be able to go through how to care for their teeth and what signs to look out for that may identify oral health problems. Try to make this a fun experience to limit anxiety around it in future. You can even bring your baby to your appointments so they feel reassured that it's a safe and friendly environment.

TEETHING: A TIRED MAMMA'S SUMMARY

Signs and symptoms of teething: include increased drooling, gnawing behaviour, ear pulling, flushed cheeks, irritability, disrupted sleep and swollen, tender gums.

Methods to alleviate teething discomfort: include gum massage, teething toys/rings, cool and soft foods, drool protection and pain relief options like paracetamol and ibuprofen.

Caring for a baby's teeth: oral health is important for tooth alignment, spacing, speech and eating. Proper toothbrushing techniques with age-appropriate toothpaste and toothbrushes should be utilised as soon as the first tooth comes in.

Tricks to make toothbrushing enjoyable: trying different toothpaste flavours, giving the baby control, using distraction techniques, singing toothbrushing songs and allowing the baby to brush their own teeth under supervision.

Dentist: schedule the baby's first dentist appointment upon the emergence of the first tooth.

CHAPTER 11

BABY VACCINATIONS

BABY'S HERE

The topic of vaccinations can be divisive, but undeniably they have played a crucial role in protecting newborns and infants from serious diseases. Newborns have an immature immune system, which leaves them vulnerable to infections. In the first few months, the mother's antibodies help to protect them, but after that the protection wears off. Vaccinations strengthen their immune response against preventable diseases and contribute to herd immunity, which safeguards those who cannot receive vaccines, usually for medical reasons.

THE UK VACCINATION SCHEDULE

In the UK, we begin routine immunisations from two months of age[198]. Ideally, you need to stick to this schedule to protect your child best, but if anything happens to delay or interrupt the schedule, don't panic; just pick it up again as soon as you can. I have included the schedule below until the age of 1, though there are more after this age.

Age	Disease	Vaccine	Route	Trade name
8 weeks	Diphtheria, tetanus, pertussis (whooping cough), polio, Haemophilus influenzae type b (Hib) and hepatitis B	DTaP/IPV/Hib/HepB Known as the 6-in-1	Injection to thigh	Infanrix hexa Or Vaxelis

Age	Disease	Vaccine	Route	Trade name
8 weeks	Meningococcal group B (MenB)	MenB	Injection to left thigh	Bexsero
	Rotavirus gastroenteritis	Rotavirus	By mouth	Rotarix
12 weeks	Diphtheria, tetanus, pertussis (whooping cough), polio, Haemophilus influenzae type b (Hib) and hepatitis B	DTaP/IPV/ Hib/HepB Known as the 6-in-1	Injection to thigh	Infanrix hexa Or Vaxelis
	Pneumococcal	PCV	Injection to thigh	Prevenar 13
	Rotavirus gastroenteritis	Rotavirus	By mouth	Rotarix
16 weeks	Diphtheria, tetanus, pertussis (whooping cough), polio, Haemophilus influenzae type b (Hib) and hepatitis B	DTaP/IPV/ Hib/HepB Known as the 6-in-1	Injection to thigh	Infanrix hexa Or Vaxelis
	Meningococcal group B (MenB)	MenB	Injection to left thigh	Bexsero
1 year	Hib and Meningococcal group C (MenC)	Hib/MenC	Injection to upper arm/thigh	Mentorix
	Pneumococcal	PCV booster	Injection to upper arm/thigh	Prevenar 13
	Measles, mumps and rubella (German measles)	MMR	Injection to upper arm/thigh	MMRvaxPro or Priorix
	Meningococcal group B (MenB)	MenB booster	Injection to left thigh	Bexsero

If you are in an area of the country where the incidence of tuberculosis is greater than 40/10,000, or your baby has a parent or grandparent born in a country with a high rate of TB, or your baby lives with or is in close contact with someone with infectious TB, your baby will also be offered the BCG vaccination. This is often offered at the hospital before you are discharged, but it can be any time after. You can find the immunisation record of your baby in the Red Book (see page xx), but if you need clarification on whether your baby has had an immunisation, you can also ask your GP.

VACCINE SIDE-EFFECTS

Most vaccinations are well tolerated, but, as with all medicines, there can be side-effects, though they are often mild. The side effects usually only last 2 or 3 days and commonly include:

Mild pain/discomfort – your baby may cry for a little while, but that usually settles soon with a cuddle or a feed.

Reaction at the injection site – they might develop some swelling, redness or a small hard lump where the injection was given, and it may be sore to touch.

Fever – these are quite common in young children but are usually low-grade and mild. It is a normal response of your baby's immune system mounting protection against the disease, though it may make your baby more irritable and uncomfortable.

Severe allergic reactions (anaphylaxis) are extremely rare. If your baby develops any breathing difficulty, hives, swelling of the face or throat, or a high fever, seek medical immediate attention.

Special notes should be made of the MenB and the MMR vaccines. Fevers are prevalent with the MenB vaccine (2 and 4 months), and you should give your baby paracetamol as soon as possible after their two- and four-month vaccinations[199]. You can give them a second dose 4–6 hours after that and a third dose 4–6 hours after that. If you have any queries, the nurse doing the injection can give you more information.

The MMR comprises three different vaccines (measles, mumps and rubella), and each can cause reactions at different times after the injection. After 6 to 10 days, the measles vaccine may cause a fever, a measles-like rash and loss of appetite. I erroneously managed to time this with Harris' first birthday party and had a pretty miserable kid on my hands, so beware! The mumps vaccine may cause mumps-like symptoms with fever and swollen glands 2 to 3 weeks after the injection. A rash and possibly a slightly raised temperature may occur 12–14 days after the rubella vaccine, but a rash may also rarely occur up to 6 weeks later.

VACCINE SAFETY

Vaccines go through a stringent process before they can be introduced. They must be licensed by the Medicines and Healthcare products Regulatory Agency (MHRA), which assesses their safety and efficacy, and their safety continues to be constantly monitored so that any new side-effects are quickly noticed and investigated.

Sadly, many myths are circulating about vaccinations, and the 'Wakefield effect' still impacts public confidence in vaccination. This term refers to the consequence of the controversial research study in 1998 by Dr Andrew Wakefield, which claimed to find a link between the MMR vaccine and autism in children. However, in the years following the publication, subsequent studies failed to replicate any findings suggesting a causal link between MMR and autism[200]. Furthermore, it was revealed that Dr Wakefield had financial motives and conflicts of interest.

The scientific community discredited the study, and the paper was retracted in 2010, and the General Medical Council (GMC) struck off Dr Wakefield. Despite this and subsequent research all showing the safety of the vaccines, doubts were sown, and it is thought that this effect signified the critical moment in vaccine hesitancy and the anti-vaccine movement. If you have any concerns about vaccine safety, it is always best to address this with your GP, who can discuss the benefits versus risks of vaccines. You can also review the MHRA website, which has the latest information on the safety of vaccines.

WHAT CAN YOU DO TO MAKE THE VACCINATION PROCESS EASIER?

I have always given Harris every available vaccination. I understand the robust safety and efficacy trials they must go through before they are deemed safe, and I also recognise that most of these vaccinations have been around for decades and have saved thousands of lives. However, I am still human and a mother, and I know that feeling of dread that greets us all when it is vaccination time. I hate the thought of purposely inflicting pain on my child (albeit momentary), and that look he gives me when he thinks I have betrayed the mother–child sanctity. Yet, I know that these short-term pains give him long-term gains, and we persevere. There are, however, some tricks that might make the process easier.

Distract – there are many ways to distract a baby, but it may come from singing, noisy rattle toys, books, blowing bubbles, pulling funny faces, gentle massage or screen time.

Swaddle – if your baby relaxes when they are swaddled, try this during and after the vaccine so that they are soothed. Just remember to keep the thighs free for the vaccine.

Feed – breastfed babies can be fed during or shortly after the immunisations to offer comfort and pain relief. A systematic review and meta-analysis[201] found that breastfeeding during immunisation reduces distress during the procedure, as well as aiding distress recovery. A Cochrane review[202] found that breastfeeding reduced pain scores and cry time, and was more effective than cuddling, sugar water or even topical anaesthetic cream.

Hold close – the most comforting place in the world for your baby is close to you, so hold them against you, offering skin-to-skin contact if possible.

Stay calm – your baby will sense your apprehension, and they regulate their emotions with you, so try to stay as positive and calm as possible. If you have any concerns about the immunisations, it is best to address these beforehand so that the process is quick, smooth and easy.

Dress appropriately – in babies under 12 months, the injections are in the thigh, so dress them in clothes that give you easy access to the thighs, avoiding the faff and distress that many babies experience when having to get undressed.

VACCINATIONS: A TIRED MAMMA'S SUMMARY

Role of vaccinations: vaccinations strengthen a baby's immune response against preventable illnesses, contributing not only to their protection but also to the concept of herd immunity.

The UK vaccination schedule: beginning at 2 months of age and continuing throughout the first year. The schedule includes various vaccines targeting diseases such as diphtheria, tetanus, pertussis, polio, hepatitis B, meningococcal group B, pneumococcal infections, rotavirus gastroenteritis, and measles, mumps and rubella. The BCG vaccine for tuberculosis is also mentioned if certain risk factors are present.

Vaccine side-effects: most are mild and short-lived, including mild pain, swelling at the injection site and low-grade fevers. Severe allergic reactions are rare but should be recognised and addressed promptly.

Tips to ease the vaccination process: include distraction techniques, swaddling, feeding, skin-to-skin contact, maintaining calm and dressing appropriately for easy access during injections.

CHAPTER 12

MILESTONES BABY'S HERE

The first year of your baby's life is incredible and full of growth and development. They progress from helpless (but cute), squishy, newborn potatoes to mischievous, fun, curious and active infants. There are many milestones along the way that mark these advancements, and observing and supporting these achievements as a parent is so fulfilling. Babies are all unique and may hit these milestones at different times, but it can be helpful to have a general framework. If you have any concerns regarding their milestones, you can discuss this with your health visitor or GP.

I often grappled throughout that first year of parenthood with a pervasive feeling that I wasn't doing enough with Harris. You are navigating uncharted territory, facing sleepless nights, the infinite nappy changes and feeds, and quite frankly managing boredom, but in the midst of this whirlwind, self-doubt tends to creep in. It is hard not to question whether you are offering enough for your baby's development, but I want to reassure you that the fact that you're even questioning it, probably means you are! Babies do not need much, and you don't have to fork out for expensive toys or go to classes to stimulate them. In fact, many of the everyday tasks you do with them are likely to be a form of play, education and development. I have added a few suggestions against each milestone category, to give you some ideas, but to also put your mind at rest that nothing extravagant is necessary.

0-1 MONTHS

The milestones in these first moments may seem basic, but these instinctive reflexes play a crucial role in your baby's survival.

- Instinctively seek food, warmth and comfort.
- Recognise caregivers' voices.
- Develop a strong bond through eye contact and touch.
- Reflexes like sucking, swallowing and grasping.

PLAY IDEAS

Tummy time can be started from birth. It is required to help them develop their neck and upper body muscles, but also gives the baby a different perspective. It is often easier to start them off by resting them on your chest and when they seem ready, migrating to the floor. It's normal for some babies not to enjoy tummy time at first, but start with a short time and gradually increase it as they get used to it. Always watch your baby during tummy time.

Gentle touch, massage and tickles are all ways to develop their sense of touch, and to offer a soothing way to bond.

Their vision is still developing, but if you have any high contrast (like black and white) images or objects, they may enjoy the patterns. I had a leopard-print muslin that did the trick with Harris.

2-3 MONTHS

During the second and third months, the baby gains more strength in their neck and upper body muscles. They also become more socially responsive.

- Start to lift their head and chest during tummy time and turn their head to the side.

- On their backs, they will wiggle and squirm, waving their arms and legs.
- They can hold a toy that you put in their hands.
- They can follow an object with both eyes, and eye-to-eye contact is deliberately maintained.
- Start cooing and making sounds when you talk to them.
- Smile when spoken to and sees familiar faces.
- Turn to voices.

PLAY IDEAS

If you have a baby gym with hanging toys for your baby to reach out for and bat, this can be an easy way to get a few minutes of peace whilst still stimulating them. We had second-hand ones (everyone wants to get rid of their bulky baby gym once their child is old enough!) but you can also make them yourself by hanging appropriate toys on a sturdy frame.

Develop their sense of hearing by playing music and dancing with them in your arms, or sing them a song. Shake rattles and show them how different objects make different sounds when you gently bang them.

Sit with them in front of a mirror, whilst they explore their reflection. Make faces, smile, poke out your tongue.

4–5 MONTHS

You can expect a significant leap in their motor skills as they reach this age, and as they explore their surroundings, they become increasingly interactive and expressive.

- They can hold their head straight up when on their tummy and look around.
- When on their back, they bring their hands together and touch their fingers.
- When sitting, they can hold their head steady without support.

- They can start to reach out for a close-by toy when sitting, and when the toy is in their hand, they will 'play' with it by looking at it, waving it about and chewing it.
- They will smile and coo at themselves in the mirror.
- They will start to laugh or softly chuckle and make high-pitched squeals.
- They will get excited to see you if you have been out of sight.
- They will make sounds when looking for toys or people.

PLAY IDEAS

Pimp up tummy time by adding props like soft toys and textured cushions for them to reach out to and play with.

Play peek-a-boo games to reinforce object permanence (but mainly because it makes them laugh). You can use nappy changing time to play these face-to-face games.

Read board books with simple pictures and bright colours. Baby sessions in the library are a fun way of exploring different books, with various pop-outs and textures.

6-7 MONTHS

Both improved physical stability and vocal abilities make these months fun to observe and encourage.

- Roll from their back to their tummy.
- Sit up with support.
- Get into a crawling position.
- Grasp a toy with one or both hands and pass it to the other hand.
- Reach a small object with a finger.
- Play with their feet when lying on their back.
- Hold up hands to be lifted.
- Can make sounds like 'da', 'ga', 'ka.'
- Laughs and squeals.
- Enjoys looking at themselves in the mirror.

PLAY IDEAS

Sing interactive songs like pat-a-cake and row your boat, and take turns clapping your hands and their hands together. Clapping requires fine-motor skills, muscle control and hand–eye coordination, so it can be a tricky milestone to achieve, but making it fun with songs can help.

Give them a sensory ball to explore with their hands and mouth. Then roll it back and forth to encourage them to reach out for it and encourage crawling movements.

Blow bubbles for them whilst sitting with them on the floor. They can track the bubbles and try to reach out for them to pop.

8–9 MONTHS

They really start to get more active from here on, and their mobility will be a new adventure.

- Pick up smaller objects with finger and thumb (pincer grip).
- Sit up without support.
- May start crawling.
- Pull themselves up to stand.
- Steadier on their feet when standing.
- Roll from their tummy to their back.
- Recognise simple commands 'give to me', and words like 'bye bye'.
- Continue to experiment with babbling and simple sounds. You may even get a 'mama'.

PLAY IDEAS

Try finger painting with safe, non-toxic paints. I used blended beetroot to make a deep purple paint and added yoghurt to make it more pink. Half of it would end up in Harris' mouth, but I took this as a nutritional bonus.

Make an obstacle course in your living room out of cushions and boxes to encourage their mobility.

Use stacking cups or nesting boxes for tactile play and problem-solving and they inevitably bring a lot of joy when they are knocked down.

10–12 MONTHS

As the first year with your new addition comes to an end, they will discover a new sense of confidence and independence, and improved communication will bring deeper connections.

- Begin 'cruising' by holding onto furniture and walking.
- Stand independently.
- Crawl and bottom shuffle.
- After pulling themselves up to stand, they can also sit back down again.
- Hand you objects.
- Create more meaningful sounds like 'Mama' and 'Dada'.
- Respond to their name.

PLAY IDEAS

Explore nature with them, in the garden or in a park. Pick up leaves, scrunch them, watch ants crawl up trees and listen out for bird song.

Puzzle play with shape sorters, building blocks and more complex stacking toys.

Role play with your baby, giving them phones (old ones, they will be dropped! Or better yet toy ones), safe kitchen utensils or dolls to imitate you.

As you can see, milestones cover many areas, including cognitive, motor, language, social and emotional development. However, they are not limited to the above, nor are they expected to occur across all these areas in the exact timeframes suggested. Understanding these milestones can help you set realistic expectations for your child's development, gauge your child's overall growth and functioning, and consider whether areas require extra attention. If you or your healthcare professional have any developmental concerns, then early intervention is best to provide the necessary support and resources to help your baby reach their full potential.

MILESTONES: A TIRED MAMMA'S SUMMARY

0-1 months: newborns instinctively seek nourishment, warmth and comfort. They bond through eye contact and touch, and exhibit reflexes like sucking and grasping.

2-3 months: babies gain strength in their neck and upper body muscles. They lift their head during tummy time, coo and make sounds, smile at familiar faces and follow objects with their eyes.

4-5 months: motor skills progress significantly, and babies become more interactive. They can hold their head up, reach for and play with toys, laugh or chuckle and show excitement when familiar faces return.

6-7 months: improved physical stability and vocal abilities emerge. Babies roll over, sit with support, get into crawling positions, grasp objects and experiment with sounds.

8-9 months: babies become more active, pick up objects with finger and thumb, sit without support, start crawling and pull themselves up to stand. Their communication skills also improve.

10-12 months: in the final months of the first year, babies begin cruising and walking with support, stand independently, crawl or shuffle and respond to their name. Communication becomes more meaningful with sounds like 'Mama' and 'Dada'.

FINAL WORD

I love Harris more than anything, and there is nothing I wouldn't do to keep him feeling safe. But parenting is the hardest job you'll ever love. I'm a doctor. I have had sleepless nights, weeks of not seeing my friends and family, the responsibility of human life in my hands, days fuelled only by caffeine, nights of crying and sheer panic. I love my job as a doctor; it is also incredibly challenging, I wouldn't swap it for anything else. Yet there are days when I have found motherhood harder.

One minute you are staring at your child wondering how you managed to create something so perfect. The next minute you are being screamed at because you couldn't find a purple-coloured apple. Despite the rollercoaster, the anxiety, the sleeplessness and the tremendous responsibility, motherhood is one of the most remarkable aspects of human existence. It is a testament to the strength, resilience and nurture of women.

In fact, being Harris' mother was so special to me that I wanted to do it all over again, and whilst writing this book, I had incredible news that I was pregnant again. I had the opportunity to write this book, going through it all first-hand again. I didn't have to search back in my memories for the antenatal journey, the highs and lows, the fears and worries of inadequacy. I wrote this, living each experience.

I am writing this final chapter while sitting in Queen Charlotte's Maternity Hospital, nearly 28 weeks pregnant, and waiting on my glucose tolerance test. Big bumps in the waiting room surround me, and I am filled with so much love and admiration for all these women. Our ability to create and nurture a child is nothing short of awe-inspiring.

The entire process, from conception and pregnancy to childbirth and motherhood, involves the intricate weaving of biological processes and a unique and powerful connection that profoundly influences your child's emotional and physical wellbeing.

As I embarked on this path of motherhood and writing this book, I couldn't help but reflect on the woman who shaped me into who I am today – my own mother. She was a shining light, my comfort, my joy, my strength and my pillar of support. Holding Harris in my arms and carrying this bump, I can't help but wonder how my mum felt on the day I was born. Did we have the same fears and aspirations as her? Have we had the same mothering style? Would I be as compassionate, caring and patient as she?

I wished my mother was still well enough to be by my side a million times in this journey, helping me through this and answering my panicked calls and texts. But I have found myself instinctively replicating my mother's practices, singing the same songs she sang me, giving the same head massages she gave me and saying the exact phrases that used to comfort me. She is with me, even when she is not.

In becoming a mother, I appreciate my own mother even more. I recognise the sacrifices she made, the challenges she faced, and the unconditional love she surrounded me with. So, to all those hopeful mammas, big- and small-bumped mammas, and brand new mammas, you are a miracle, you will be the best mother that you can be, and you are good enough.

ENDNOTES

1. NHS Infertility Overview, 2020, www.nhs.uk/conditions/infertility/
2. Pitkin RM. Folate and neural tube defects. Am J Clin Nutr. 2007 Jan;85(1):285S–288S. doi: 10.1093/ajcn/85.1.285S.
3. Hollowell J, Pillas D, Rowe R, Linsell L, Knight M, Brocklehurst P. The impact of maternal obesity on intrapartum outcomes in otherwise low risk women: secondary analysis of the Birthplace national prospective cohort study. BJOG. 2014 Feb;121(3):343–55. doi: 10.1111/1471-0528.12437.
4. NHS, Pregnancy, breastfeeding and fertility while taking or using ibuprofen, 2021 https://www.nhs.uk/medicines/ibuprofen-for-adults /pregnancy-breastfeeding-and-fertility-while-taking-ibuprofen/
5. Ried K, Stuart K. Efficacy of traditional Chinese herbal medicine in the management of female infertility: a systematic review. Complement Ther Med. 2011 Dec;19(6):319–31. doi: 10.1016/j.ctim.2011.09.003.
6. Yun L, Liqun W, Shuqi Y, Chunxiao W, Liming L, Wei Y. Acupuncture for infertile women without undergoing assisted reproductive techniques (ART): a systematic review and meta-analysis. Medicine (Baltimore). 2019 Jul;98(29):e16463. doi: 10.1097/MD.0000000000016463.
7. Peng T, Yin LL, Xiong Y, Xie F, Ji CY, Yang Z, Pan Q, Li MQ, Deng XD, Dong J, Wu JN. Maternal traditional Chinese medicine exposure and risk of congenital malformations: a multicenter prospective cohort study. Acta Obstet Gynecol Scand. 2023 Jun;102(6):735–743. doi: 10.1111 /aogs.14553.
8. Ondrizek RR, Chan PJ, Patton WC, King A. An alternative medicine study of herbal effects on the penetration of zona-free hamster oocytes and the integrity of sperm deoxyribonucleic acid. Fertil Steril. 1999 Mar;71(3): 517–22. doi: 10.1016/s0015-0282(98)00476-2.
9. Daw JR, Hanley GE, Greyson DL, Morgan SG. Prescription drug use during pregnancy in developed countries: a systematic review.

Pharmacoepidemiol Drug Saf. 2011 Sep;20(9):895–902. doi: 10.1002 /pds.2184.

10. Pryor J, Patrick SW, Sundermann AC, Wu P, Hartmann KE. Pregnancy intention and maternal alcohol consumption. Obstet Gynecol. 2017;129:727–733. doi: 10.1097/AOG.0000000000001933.

11. Emanuele MA, Wezeman F, Emanuele NV. Alcohol's effects on female reproductive function. Alcohol Res Heal. 2002;26:274–281.

12. Van Heertum K, Rossi B. Alcohol and fertility: how much is too much? Fertil Res Pract. 2017 Jul 10;3:10. doi: 10.1186/s40738-017-0037-x.

13. Jensen TK, Hjollund HI, Henriksen TB, Scheike T, Kolstad H, Giwercman A, et al. Does moderate alcohol consumption affect fertility? Follow-up study among couples planning first pregnancy. BMJ. 1998;317.

14. Juhl M, Andersen A-MN, Grønbaek M, Olsen J. Moderate alcohol consumption and waiting time to pregnancy. Hum Reprod. 2002;16: 2705–2709. doi: 10.1093/humrep/16.12.2705.

15. Rooney KL, Domar AD. The relationship between stress and infertility. Dialogues Clin Neurosci. 2018 Mar;20(1):41–47. doi: 10.31887/DCNS .2018.20.1/klrooney.

16. Nykjaer C, Alwan NA, Greenwood DC, Simpson NA, Hay AW, White KL, Cade JE. Maternal alcohol intake prior to and during pregnancy and risk of adverse birth outcomes: evidence from a British cohort. J Epidemiol Community Health. 2014 Jun;68(6):542–549. doi: 10.1136/jech-2013 -202934.

17. FSRH, The mental health impact of unplanned pregnancy and the right to abortion https://www.fsrh.org/blogs/the-mental-health-impact-for-all -with-unplanned-pregnancy-and/

18. NHS, Sleep problems https://www.nhs.uk/every-mind-matters/mental -health-issues/sleep/

19. Institute of Medicine (US) Committee on Military Nutrition Research. Caffeine for the sustainment of mental task performance: formulations for military operations. Washington (DC): National Academies Press (US); 2001. 2, Pharmacology of Caffeine.

20. Einarson TR, Piwko C, Koren G. Quantifying the global rates of nausea and vomiting of pregnancy: a meta analysis. J Popul Ther Clin Pharmacol. 2013;20(2):e171–e183.

21. Lee NM, Saha S. Nausea and vomiting of pregnancy. Gastroenterol Clin North Am. 2011 Jun;40(2):309–334, vii. doi: 10.1016/j.gtc.2011.03.009.

22. Sridharan K, Sivaramakrishnan G. Interventions for treating nausea and vomiting in pregnancy: a network meta-analysis and trial sequential

analysis of randomized clinical trials. Expert Rev Clin Pharmacol. 2018 Nov;11(11):1143–1150. doi: 10.1080/17512433.2018.1530108.

23. Lete I, Allué J. The effectiveness of ginger in the prevention of nausea and vomiting during pregnancy and chemotherapy. Integr Med Insights. 2016 Mar 31;11:11–17. doi: 10.4137/IMI.S36273.

24. https://www.rcog.org.uk/media/y3fen1x1/gtg69-hyperemesis.pdf

25. National Institute for Health and Care and Excellence. Doxylamine/pyridoxine (Xonvea) for treating nausea and vomiting of pregnancy, 2019 https://www.nice.org.uk/advice/es20/chapter/key-messages

26. NHS, Water, drinks and hydration https://www.nhs.uk/live-well/eat-well/food-guidelines-and-food-labels/water-drinks-nutrition/

27. Sahakian V, Rouse D, Sipes S, Rose N, Niebyl J. Vitamin B6 is effective therapy for nausea and vomiting of pregnancy: a randomized, double-blind placebo-controlled study. Obstet Gynecol. 1991 Jul;78(1):33–36.

28. American College of Obstetricians and Gynaecologists, Morning sickness: nausea and vomiting of pregnancy, 2020 https://www.acog.org/womens-health/faqs/morning-sickness-nausea-and-vomiting-of-pregnancy

29. Orloff NC, Hormes JM. Pickles and ice cream! Food cravings in pregnancy: hypotheses, preliminary evidence, and directions for future research. Front Psychol. 2014 Sep 23;5:1076. doi: 10.3389/fpsyg.2014.01076.

30. Caparroz FA, Gregorio LL, Bongiovanni G, Izu SC, Kosugi EM. Rhinitis and pregnancy: literature review. Braz J Otorhinolaryngol. 2016 Jan–Feb; 82(1):105–111. doi: 10.1016/j.bjorl.2015.04.011.

31. Gov.UK, Pregnancy: advice on contact with animals that area giving birth, 2017 https://www.gov.uk/guidance/pregnancy-advice-on-contact-with-animals-that-are-giving-birth

32. NHS, Toxoplasmosis, 2023 https://www.nhs.uk/conditions/toxoplasmosis/

33. NHS, Foods to avoid in pregnancy, 2023 https://www.nhs.uk/pregnancy/keeping-well/foods-to-avoid/

34. Centers for Disease Control and Prevention, Weight gain during pregnancy, 2023 https://www.cdc.gov/reproductivehealth/maternalinfanthealth/pregnancy-weight-gain.htm

35. Royal College of Obstetricians and Gynaecologists, Recreational exercise and pregnancy patient information leaflet, 2016 https://www.rcog.org.uk/for-the-public/browse-all-patient-information-leaflets/recreational-exercise-and-pregnancy-patient-information-leaflet/

36. Gupta R, Dhyani M, Kendzerska T, Pandi-Perumal SR, BaHammam AS, Srivanitchapoom P, Pandey S, Hallett M. Restless legs syndrome and

pregnancy: prevalence, possible pathophysiological mechanisms and treatment. Acta Neurol Scand. 2016 May;133(5):320–329. doi: 10.1111 /ane.12520.

37. NHS, Reducing the risk of stillbirth, 2021 https://www.nhs.uk /pregnancy/keeping-well/reducing-the-risk-of-stillbirth/

38. Stacey T, Thompson JMD, Mitchell EA, Ekeroma AJ, Zuccollo JM, McCowan LME, et al. Association between maternal sleep practices and risk of late stillbirth: a case-control study. BMJ 2011;342:d3403. doi:10.1136/bmj.d3403.

39. Gordon A, Raynes-Greenow C, Bond D, Morris J, Rawlinson W, Jeffery H. Sleep position, fetal growth restriction, and late-pregnancy stillbirth: the Sydney stillbirth study. Obstet Gynecol. 2015 Feb;125(2):347–355. doi: 10.1097/AOG.0000000000000627.

40. Platts J, Mitchell EA, Stacey T, et al. The Midland and North of England Stillbirth Study (MiNESS). BMC Pregnancy Childbirth 14, 171 (2014). https://doi.org/10.1186/1471-2393-14-171

41. Tommy's. Stillbirth statistics https://www.tommys.org/baby-loss-support /stillbirth-information-and-support/stillbirth-statistics

42. Stone P R, Burgess W, McIntyre J, Gunn AJ, Lear CA, Bennet L, Mitchell EA, Thompson JMD. An investigation of fetal behavioural states during maternal sleep in healthy late gestation pregnancy: an observational study. The JOP, 2017; doi: 10.1113/JP275084.

43. Silver RM, Hunter S, Reddy UM, Facco F, Gibbins KJ, Grobman WA, Mercer BM, Haas DM, Simhan HN, Parry S, Wapner RJ, Louis J, Chung JM, Pien G, Schubert FP, Saade GR, Zee P, Redline S, Parker CB. Nulliparous pregnancy outcomes study: monitoring mothers-to-be (numom2b) study. Prospective evaluation of maternal sleep position through 30 weeks of gestation and adverse pregnancy outcomes. Obstet Gynecol. 2019 Oct;134(4):667–676. doi: 10.1097/AOG.000000000000 3458.

44. Dugas C, Slane VH. Miscarriage. 2022 Jun 27. In: StatPearls [Internet]. Treasure Island (FL): StatPearls Publishing; 2023 Jan–.

45. NHS, 11 physical conditions (20-week scan) 2022 https://www.gov.uk /government/publications/screening-tests-for-you-and-your-baby/11 -physical-conditions-20-week-scan

46. van Nisselrooij AEL, Teunissen AKK, Clur SA, Rozendaal L, Pajkrt E, Linskens IH, Rammeloo L, van Lith JMM, Blom NA, Haak MC. Why are congenital heart defects being missed? Ultrasound Obstet Gynecol. 2020 Jun;55(6):747–757. doi: 10.1002/uog.20358.

47. Royal College of Obstetricians & Gynaecologists. Amniocentesis and chorionic villus sampling (Green-top Guideline No. 8), 2021 https://www .rcog.org.uk/guidance/browse-all-guidance/green-top-guidelines /amniocentesis-and-chorionic-villus-sampling-green-top-guideline-no-8/

48. Royal College of Obstetricians & Gynaecologists. COVID-19 vaccines, pregnancy and breastfeeding FAQs https://www.rcog.org.uk/guidance /coronavirus-covid-19-pregnancy-and-women-s-health/vaccination/covid -19-vaccines-pregnancy-and-breastfeeding-faqs/

49. Royal College of Obstetricians & Gynaecologists. Treatment of venous thrombosis in pregnancy and after birth patient information leaflet https://www.rcog.org.uk/for-the-public/browse-all-patient-information -leaflets/treatment-of-venous-thrombosis-in-pregnancy-and-after-birth -patient-information-leaflet/

50. National Institute for Health and Care Excellence. Hypertension in pregnancy, 2022 https://cks.nice.org.uk/topics/hypertension-in-pregnancy /background-information/prevalence/

51. Royal College of Obstetricians & Gynaecologists. Intrahepatic cholestasis of pregnancy, 2022 https://www.rcog.org.uk/for-the-public/browse-all -patient-information-leaflets/intrahepatic-cholestasis-of-pregnancy-patient -information-leaflet/

52. Royal College of Obstetricians and Gynaecologists. Intrahepatic cholestasis of pregnancy, 2022 https://www.rcog.org.uk/for-the-public/browse-all -patient-information-leaflets/intrahepatic-cholestasis-of-pregnancy-patient -information-leaflet/

53. Royal College of Obstetricians & Gynaecologists. Pregnancy sickness (nausea and vomiting of pregnancy and hyperemesis gravidarum) https:// www.rcog.org.uk/for-the-public/browse-all-patient-information-leaflets /pregnancy-sickness-nausea-and-vomiting-of-pregnancy-and-hyperemesis -gravidarum/

54. Miscarriage Association. Background information: miscarriage, 2021. https://bit.ly/3HE5zxa (accessed 27 December 2021)

55. Royal College of Obstetricians and Gynaecologists. Placenta praevia, placenta accreta and vasa praevia, 2018 https://www.rcog.org.uk /globalassets/documents/patients/patient-information-leaflets/pregnancy /pi-placenta-praevia-placenta-accreta-and-vasa-praevia.pdf

56. Tikkanen M. Placental abruption: epidemiology, risk factors and consequences. Acta Obstetricia et Gynecologica Scandinavica, 90: 140–149.

57. Royal College of Obstetricians and Gynaecologists. Placenta praevia, placenta accreta and vasa praevia, 2018 https://www.rcog.org.uk

/globalassets/documents /patients/patient-information-leaflets/pregnancy /pi-placenta-praevia-placenta-accreta-and-vasa-praevia.pdf

58. Royal College of Obstetricians and Gynaecologists. Group B Streptococcus (GBS) in pregnancy and newborn babies https://www.rcog.org.uk/for -the-public/browse-all-patient-information-leaflets/group-b-streptococcus -gbs-in-pregnancy-and-newborn-babies/

59. Muller-Pebody B, Johnson AP, Heath PT, et al. Empirical treatment of neonatal sepsis: are the current guidelines adequate? Arch Dis Child Fetal Neonatal Ed. 2011; 96:F4–F8.

60. Stephens K, Charnock-Jones DS, Smith GCS. Group B Streptococcus and the risk of perinatal morbidity and mortality following term labor. Am J Obstet Gynecol. 2023 May;228(5S):S1305–S1312. doi: 10.1016/j .ajog.2022.07.051.

61. Bevan D, White A, Marshall J, Peckham C. Modelling the effect of the introduction of antenatal screening for group B Streptococcus (GBS) carriage in the UK. BMJ Open. 2019; 9e024324.

62. Stephens K, Charnock-Jones DS, Smith GCS. Group B Streptococcus and the risk of perinatal morbidity and mortality following term labor. Am J Obstet Gynecol. 2023 May;228(5S):S1305–S1312. doi: 10.1016/j .ajog.2022.07.051.

63. NCT, Birth options – planning where to give birth https://www.nct.org.uk /labour-birth/getting-ready-for-birth/birth-options-planning-where-give-birth

64. Madden K, Middleton P, Cyna AM, Matthewson M, Jones L. Hypnosis for pain management during labour and childbirth. Cochrane Database of Systematic Reviews 2016, Issue 5. Art. No.: CD009356. DOI: 10.1002 /14651858.CD009356.pub3.

65. Moghaddam Hosseini V, Nazarzadeh M, Jahanfar S. Interventions for reducing fear of childbirth: a systematic review and meta-analysis of clinical trials. Women Birth. 2018 Aug;31(4):254–262. doi: 10.1016/j .wombi.2017.10.007.

66. Finlayson K, Downe S, Hinder S, Carr H, Spiby H, Whorwell P. Unexpected consequences: women's experiences of a self-hypnosis intervention to help with pain relief during labour. BMC Pregnancy Childbirth. 2015 Sep 25;15:229. doi: 10.1186/s12884-015-0659-0.

67. National Institute for Health and Care Excellence, Intrapartum care for healthy women and babies, 2023 https://www.nice.org.uk/guidance/ng235

68. Wszolek, K. Hand expressing in pregnancy and colostrum harvesting – Preparation for successful breastfeeding? BJM 2015. doi: 10.12968/bjom .2015.23.4.268

69. Frohlich J, Kettle C. Perineal care. BMJ Clin Evid. 2015 Mar 10;2015:1401.

70. Perineal massage in the weeks leading up to delivery helps some women avoid episiotomy. BMJ. 2006 Mar 18;332(7542):0.

71. Beckmann MM, Stock OM. Antenatal perineal massage for reducing perineal trauma. Cochrane Database Syst Rev. 2013 Apr 30;(4):CD005123. doi: 10.1002/14651858.CD005123.pub3.

72. Woodley SJ, Boyle R, Cody JD, Mørkved S, Hay-Smith EJC. Pelvic floor muscle training for prevention and treatment of urinary and faecal incontinence in antenatal and postnatal women. Cochrane Database Syst Rev. 2017 Dec 22;12(12):CD007471. doi: 10.1002/14651858. CD007471.pub3. Update in: Cochrane Database Syst Rev. 2020 May 6;5:CD007471.

73. Khambalia AZ, Roberts CL, Nguyen M, Algert CS, Nicholl MC, Morris J. Predicting date of birth and examining the best time to date a pregnancy. Int J Gynaecol Obstet. 2013 Nov;123(2):105–109. doi: 10.1016/j.ijgo.2013.05.007.

74. Knight B, Brereton A, Powell RJ, Liversedge H. Assessing the accuracy of ultrasound estimation of gestational age during routine antenatal care in in vitro fertilization (IVF) pregnancies. Ultrasound. 2018 Feb;26(1):49–53. doi: 10.1177/1742271X17751257.

75. CDC. Births: final data for 2017 https://stacks.cdc.gov/view/cdc/60432.

76. Kordi M, Meybodi FA, Tara F, Fakari FR, Nemati M, Shakeri M. Effect of dates in late pregnancy on the duration of labor in nulliparous women. Iran J Nurs Midwifery Res. 2017 Sep-Oct;22(5):383–387. doi: 10.4103 /ijnmr.IJNMR_213_15.

77. Bowman R, Taylor J, Muggleton S, Davis D. Biophysical effects, safety and efficacy of raspberry leaf use in pregnancy: a systematic integrative review. BMC Complement Med Ther. 2021 Feb 9;21(1):56. doi: 10.1186/s12906-021-03230-4.

78. National Institute for Health and Care Excellence. Guideline: inducing labour, 2021 https://www.nice.org.uk/guidance/ng207/documents/draft -guideline-2

79. Smith CA, Armour M, Dahlen HG. Acupuncture or acupressure for induction of labour. Cochrane Database Syst Rev. 2017 Oct 17;10(10):CD002962. doi: 10.1002/14651858.CD002962.pub4.

80. Monji F, Adaikan PG, Lau LC, Bin Said B, Gong Y, Tan HM, Choolani M. Investigation of uterotonic properties of Ananas comosus extracts. J Ethnopharmacol. 2016 Dec 4;193:21–29. doi: 10.1016/j.jep.2016.07.041.

81. Yakubu MT, Olawepo OJ, Fasoranti GA. Ananas comosus: is the unripe fruit juice an abortifacient in pregnant Wistar rats? Eur J Contracept Reprod Health Care. 2011 Oct;16(5):397–402. doi: 10.3109/13625187.2011.599454.

82. Kavanagh J, Kelly AJ, Thomas J. Breast stimulation for cervical ripening and induction of labour. Cochrane Database Syst Rev. 2005 Jul 20;2005(3):CD003392. doi: 10.1002/14651858.CD003392.pub2.

83. NHS. Inducing labour, 2023 https://www.nhs.uk/pregnancy/labour-and-birth/signs-of-labour/inducing-labour/

84. National Institute for Health and Care Excellence. Inducing labour, 2021 https://www.nice.org.uk/guidance/NG207

85. Rosenstein MG, Cheng YW, Snowden JM, Nicholson JM, Caughey AB. Risk of stillbirth and infant death stratified by gestational age. Obstet Gynecol. 2012 Jul;120(1):76–82. doi: 10.1097/AOG.0b013e31825bd286.

86. Dahlen HG, Thornton C, Downe S, et al. Intrapartum interventions and outcomes for women and children following induction of labour at term in uncomplicated pregnancies: a 16-year population-based linked data study. BMJ Open 2021; 11:e047040. doi: 10.1136/bmjopen-2020-047040.

87. Seijmonsbergen-Schermers A, Peters LL, Downe S, Dahlen H, de Jonge A. Induction of labour and emergency caesarean section in English maternity services: Examining outcomes is needed before recommending changes in practice. BJOG. 2023 Apr;130(5):542–543. doi: 10.1111/1471-0528.17359.

88. National Institute for Health and Care Excellence. Induction of labour, 2008 https://www.nhs.uk/planners/pregnancycareplanner/documents/nice_induction_of_labour.pdf

89. NHS. 2019 survey of women's experiences of maternity care, 2019 https://www.cqc.org.uk/sites/default/files/20200128_mat19_statistical release.pdf

90. Zang Y, Lu H, Zhao Y, Huang J, Ren L, Li X. Effects of flexible sacrum positions during the second stage of labour on maternal and neonatal outcomes: a systematic review and meta-analysis. J Clin Nurs. 2020 Sep; 29(17–18):3154–3169. doi: 10.1111/jocn.15376.

91. NHS, Overview Caesarean section, 2023 https://www.nhs.uk/conditions/caesarean-section/

92. Royal College of Obstetricians & Gynaecologists, Considering a caesarean birth patient information leaflet, 2022 https://www.rcog.org.uk/for-the-public/browse-all-patient-information-leaflets/considering-a-caesarean-birth-patient-information-leaflet/

93. National Institute for Health and Care Excellence. Intrapartum care for healthy women and babies NICE (CG190) 2017.

94. NHS. Information for women going home with pre-labour rupture of membranes at term (PROM), 2018 https://www.hey.nhs.uk/patient-leaflet /information-women-going-home-pre-labour-rupture-membranes-term -prom/

95. Royal College of Obstetricians & Gynaecologists. Care of a third- or fourth-degree tear that occurred during childbirth, https://www.rcog.org .uk/for-the-public/browse-all-patient-information-leaflets/care-of-a-third -or-fourth-degree-tear-that-occurred-during-childbirth-also-known-as -obstetric-anal-sphincter-injury-oasi/

96. Royal College of Obstetricians & Gynaecologists. Assisted vaginal birth (ventouse or forceps), 2020 https://www.rcog.org.uk/for-the-public/browse -all-patient-information-leaflets/assisted-vaginal-birth-ventouse-or-forceps/ https://www.yorkhospitals.nhs.uk/seecmsfile/?id=7023

97. Royal College of Obstetricians & Gynaecologists. Assisted vaginal birth (ventouse or forceps), 2020 https://www.rcog.org.uk/media/2p4fh2kd/pi -vaginal-birth-final-28042020.pdf

98. Ibid.

99. Royal College of Obstetricians & Gynaecologists. Perineal tears during childbirth https://www.rcog.org.uk/for-the-public/perineal-tears-and -episiotomies-in-childbirth/perineal-tears-during-childbirth/

100. Royal College of Obstetricians & Gynaecologists. Breech baby at the end of pregnancy, 2017 https://www.rcog.org.uk/for-the-public/browse-all -patient-information-leaflets/breech-baby-at-the-end-of-pregnancy-patient -information-leaflet/

101. Watts NP, Petrovska K, Bisits A, et al. This baby is not for turning: women's experiences of attempted external cephalic version. BMC Pregnancy Childbirth 16, 248 (2016). https://doi.org/10.1186/s12884-016-1038-1

102. Maidstone and Tunbridge Wells NHS Trust, Moxibustion, 2016 http:// www.mtw.nhs.uk/wp-content/uploads/2016/11/Moxibustion-RWF-OPLF -PWC107.pdf

103. Hofmeyr GJ, Kulier R. Cephalic version by postural management for breech presentation. Cochrane Database Syst Rev. 2012 Oct 17;10(10): CD000051. doi: 10.1002/14651858.CD000051.pub2.

104. National Institute for Health and Care Excellence. Intrapartum care for healthy women and babies, 2022 https://www.nice.org.uk/guidance/cg190 /ifp/chapter/if-there-is-meconium-during-labour

105. BMJ. Best Practice, 2022 https://bestpractice.bmj.com/topics/en-gb/1117

106. Alfirevic Z, Devane D, Gyte GM, Cuthbert A. Continuous cardiotocography (CTG) as a form of electronic fetal monitoring (EFM) for fetal assessment during labour. Cochrane Database Syst Rev. 2017 Feb 3;2(2):CD006066. doi: 10.1002/14651858.CD006066.pub3.

107. National Institute for Care and Health Excellence, Indications for continuous cardiotocography monitoring in labour, 2022 https://www.nice.org.uk/guidance/ng229/chapter/Recommendations

108. Royal College of Obstetricians & Gynaecologists, Shoulder dystocia patient information leaflet, 2012 https://www.rcog.org.uk/for-the-public/browse-all-patient-information-leaflets/shoulder-dystocia-patient-information-leaflet/

109. Chen SF, Wang CH, Chan PT, Chiang HW, Hu TM, Tam KW, Loh EW. Labour pain control by aromatherapy: a meta-analysis of randomised controlled trials. Women Birth. 2019 Aug;32(4):327–335. doi: 10.1016/j.wombi.2018.09.010.

110. National Institute for Health and Care Excellence. Intrapartum care for healthy women and babies https://www.nice.org.uk/guidance/cg190/chapter/recommendations

111. Chen SF, Wang CH, Chan PT, Chiang HW, Hu TM, Tam KW, Loh EW. Labour pain control by aromatherapy: a meta-analysis of randomised controlled trials. Women Birth. 2019 Aug;32(4):327–335. doi: 10.1016/j.wombi.2018.09.010.

112. Milton Keynes University Hospital NHS Foundation Trust, Use of water in labour and birth, https://www.mkuh.nhs.uk/patient-information-leaflet/use-of-water-in-labour-and-birth-leaflet

113. Cluett ER, Burns E. Immersion in water in labour and birth. Cochrane Database Syst Rev. 2009 Apr 15;(2):CD000111. doi: 10.1002/14651858.CD000111.pub3. Update in: Cochrane Database Syst Rev. 2018 May 16;5:CD000111.

114. National Institute for Health and Care Excellence. Intrapartum care for healthy women and babies, 2014 https://www.nice.org.uk/guidance/cg190/chapter/recommendations

115. The Royal College of Anaesthetists (RCoA) and Association of Anaesthetists of Great Britain and Ireland (AAGBI). Headache after epidural or spinal injection, 2015 https://www.hdft.nhs.uk/wp-content/uploads/2016/02/headache-after-epidural-or-spinal-injection.pdf

116. The Leeds Teaching Hospitals NHS Trust. Risks of regional anaesthesia (epidurals & spinals) and general anaesthesia, 2022 https://flipbooks.leedsth.nhs.uk/LN005147.pdf

117. Emma's Diary, What is the APGAR score? Sophie Martin https://www
.emmasdiary.co.uk/baby/new-born-care/what-is-the-apgar-score

118. Widström AM, Brimdyr K, Svensson K, Cadwell K, Nissen E. Skin-to-
skin contact the first hour after birth, underlying implications and
clinical practice. Acta Paediatr. 2019 Jul;108(7):1192–1204. doi:
10.1111/apa.14754.

119. Vaglio S. Chemical communication and mother-infant recognition.
Commun Integr Biol. 2009 May;2(3):279–281. doi: 10.4161/cib.2.3.8227.

120. Shorey S, He HG, Morelius E. Skin-to-skin contact by fathers and the
impact on infant and paternal outcomes: an integrative review. Midwifery.
2016 Sep;40:207–217. doi: 10.1016/j.midw.2016.07.007.

121. WHO. Delayed clamping of the umbilical cord to reduce infant anaemia,
2012 https://apps.who.int/iris/bitstream/handle/10665/120074/WHO
_RHR_14.19_eng.pdf;jsessionid=83A9760B1DD236976992758C47
339E5E?sequence=1

122. The American College of Obstetricians and Gynecologists. Delayed
umbilical cord clamping, 2017 https://www.acog.org/clinical/clinical
-guidance/committee-opinion/articles/2020/12/delayed-umbilical-cord
-clamping-after-birth

123. Royal College of Obstetricians & Gynaecologists. Clamping of the
umbilical cord and placental transfusion (Scientific Paper No. 14), 2015
https://www.rcog.org.uk/guidance/browse-all-guidance/scientific-impact
-papers/clamping-of-the-umbilical-cord-and-placental-transfusion-scientific
-impact-paper-no-14/

124. Mercer JS, Erickson-Owens DA, Deoni SCL, Dean DC 3rd, Collins J,
Parker AB, Wang M, Joelson S, Mercer EN, Padbury JF. Effects of Delayed
cord clamping on 4-month ferritin levels, brain myelin content, and
neurodevelopment: a randomized controlled trial. J Pediatr. 2018
Dec;203:266–272.e2. doi: 10.1016/j.jpeds.2018.06.006.

125. KC, A, Målqvist M, Rana N, et al. Effect of timing of umbilical cord
clamping on anaemia at 8 and 12 months and later neurodevelopment in
late pre-term and term infants; a facility-based, randomized-controlled trial
in Nepal. BMC Pediatr 16, 35 (2016).

126. Andersson O, Hellström-Westas L, Andersson D, Domellöf M. Effect of
delayed versus early umbilical cord clamping on neonatal outcomes and
iron status at 4 months: a randomised controlled trial. BMJ. 2011 Nov
15;343:d7157. doi: 10.1136/bmj.d7157.

127. NHS. Childhood cataracts, 2022 https://www.nhs.uk/conditions
/childhood-cataracts/

128. NHS. Overview: congenital heart disease, 2021 www.nhs.uk/conditions /congenital-heart-disease/

129. McLanders K. Reducing risk of hip problems in babies, 2020 https:// phescreening.blog.gov.uk/2020/01/23/reducing-risk-of-hip-problems-in-babies/

130. NHS and Office for Health Improvement and Disparities. Eyes, heart, hips and testes (physical examination) https://www.gov.uk/government /publications/screening-tests-for-you-and-your-baby/eyes-heart-hips-and -testes-physical-examination

131. North Bristol NHS Trust. Feeding your baby https://www.nbt.nhs.uk /maternity-services/feeding-your-baby/weight-loss

132. Ghaffari P, Vanda R, Aramesh S, et al. Hospital discharge on the first compared with the second day after a planned Cesarean delivery had equivalent maternal postpartum outcomes: a randomized single-blind controlled clinical trial. BMC Pregnancy Childbirth. 2021 Jun 30;21(1):466. doi: 10.1186/s12884-021-03873-8.

133. Gov.UK. Postnatal depression https://view-health-screening-recommendations .service.gov.uk/postnatal-depression/

134. Ibid.

135. FSRH. Clinical guideline: contraception after pregnancy (January 2017, amended October 2020) https://www.fsrh.org/documents/contraception -after-pregnancy-guideline-january-2017/

136. Gutzeit O, Levy G, Lowenstein L. Postpartum female sexual function: risk factors for postpartum sexual dysfunction. Sex Med. 2020 Mar;8(1):8–13. doi: 10.1016/j.esxm.2019.10.005.

137. Ibid.

138. Malary M, Moosazadeh M, Keramat A, Sabetghadam S. Factors influencing low sexual desire and sexual distress in pregnancy: a cross-sectional study. Int J Reprod Biomed. 2021 Nov 4;19(10):909–920. doi: 10.18502/ijrm.v19i10.9823.

139. Vekemans M. Postpartum contraception: the lactational amenorrhea method. Eur J Contracept Reprod Health Care. 1997 Jun;2(2):105–111. doi: 10.3109/13625189709167463.

140. FSRH. Clinical Guideline: contraception after pregnancy (January 2017, amended October 2020) https://www.fsrh.org/standards-and-guidance /documents/contraception-after-pregnancy-guideline-january-2017/

141. NHS Sexual Health South West London. Cap or diaphragms https:// shswl.nhs.uk/contraception/cap-or-diaphragms

142. NHS Inform. Female sterilisation, 2022 https://www.nhsinform.scot /healthy-living/contraception/female-sterilisation

143. Ceydeli A, Rucinski J, Wise L. Finding the best abdominal closure: an evidence-based review of the literature. Curr Surg. 2005 Mar-Apr; 62(2):220–225. doi: 10.1016/j.cursur.2004.08.014.

144. Kar S, Krishnan A, Shivkumar PV. Pregnancy and skin. J Obstet Gynaecol India. 2012 Jun;62(3):268–275. doi: 10.1007/s13224-012 -0179-z.

145. Sharman A. Menstruation after childbirth. J Obstet Gynaecol Br Emp. 1951;58:440–445.

146. Howie PW, McNeilly AS, Houston MJ, Cook A, Boyle H. Fertility after childbirth: post-partum ovulation and menstruation in bottle and breast feeding mothers. Clin Endocrinol (Oxf). 1982 Oct;17(4):323–332. doi: 10.1111/j.1365-2265.1982.tb01597.x.

147. World Health Organisation. Infant and young child feeding: model chapter for textbooks for medical students and allied health professionals. Geneva: World Health Organisation; 2009. SESSION 2, The physiological basis of breastfeeding

148. Kent JC, Mitoulas LR, Cregan MD, Ramsay DT, Doherty DA, Hartmann PE. Volume and frequency of breastfeedings and fat content of breast milk throughout the day. Pediatrics. 2006 Mar;117(3):e387–e395. doi: 10.1542/peds.2005-1417.

149. Dieterich CM, Felice JP, O'Sullivan E, Rasmussen KM. Breastfeeding and health outcomes for the mother–infant dyad. Pediatr Clin North Am. 2013 Feb;60(1):31–48. doi: 10.1016/j.pcl.2012.09.010.

150. AlThuneyyan DA, AlGhamdi FF, AlZain RN, AlDhawyan ZS, Alhmly HF, Purayidathil TS, AlGindan YY, Abdullah AA. The effect of breastfeeding on intelligence quotient and social intelligence among seven- to nine-year-old girls: a pilot study. Front Nutr. 2022 Feb 18;9:726042. doi: 10.3389/fnut.2022.726042.

151. Chowdhury R, Sinha B, Sankar MJ, Taneja S, Bhandari N, Rollins N, Bahl R, Martines J. Breastfeeding and maternal health outcomes: a systematic review and meta-analysis. Acta Paediatr. 2015 Dec;104(467):96–113. doi: 10.1111/apa.13102.

152. Russell MW. JAHA Spotlight on pregnancy and its impact on maternal and offspring cardiovascular health. J Am Heart Assoc. 2022 Jan 18;11(2):e025167. doi: 10.1161/JAHA.121.025167.

153. Jordan SJ, Na R, Johnatty SE, Wise LA, et al. Breastfeeding and endometrial cancer risk: an analysis from the Epidemiology of Endometrial Cancer Consortium. Obstet Gynecol. 2017 Jun;129(6):1059–1067. doi: 10.1097/AOG.0000000000002057.

154. Wagner CL, Taylor SN, Johnson DD, Hollis BW. The role of vitamin D in pregnancy and lactation: emerging concepts. Womens Health (Lond). 2012 May;8(3):323–340. doi: 10.2217/whe.12.17.

155. World Health Organisation. MCA early initiation of breastfeeding https:// www.who.int/data/gho/indicator-metadata-registry/imr-details/early -initiation-of-breastfeeding-(-)

156. Ekubay M, Berhe A, Yisma E. Initiation of breastfeeding within one hour of birth among mothers with infants younger than or equal to 6 months of age attending public health institutions in Addis Ababa, Ethiopia. Int Breastfeed J. 2018 Jan 23;13:4. doi: 10.1186/s13006-018-0146-0.

157. World Health Organisation. Breastfeeding https://www.who.int/health -topics/breastfeeding

158. UNICEF. Breastfeeding in the UK https://www.unicef.org.uk /babyfriendly/about/breastfeeding-in-the-uk/

159. Royal College of Obstetricians & Gynaecologists. Alcohol and pregnancy https://www.rcog.org.uk/for-the-public/browse-all-patient-information -leaflets/alcohol-and-pregnancy/

160. La Leche League. Breastfeeding info drinking alcohol and breastfeeding, 2021 https://llli.org/breastfeeding-info/alcohol/

161. Mayo Clinic. Diaper rash, 2023 https://www.mayoclinic.org/diseases -conditions/diaper-rash/diagnosis-treatment/drc-20371641

162. Drinkaware. Alcohol and breastfeeding, 2022 https://www.drinkaware.co .uk/facts/health-effects-of-alcohol/alcohol-fertility-and-pregnancy/alcohol -and-breastfeeding

163. NHS. Breastfeeding and drinking alcohol, 2019 https://www.nhs.uk /conditions/pregnancy-and-baby/breastfeeding-alcohol/

164. Wilson J, Tay RY, McCormack C, Allsop S, Najman J, Burns L, Olsson CA, Elliott E, Jacobs S, Mattick RP, Hutchinson D. Alcohol consumption by breastfeeding mothers: frequency, correlates and infant outcomes. Drug Alcohol Rev. 2017 Sep;36(5):667–676. doi: 10.1111/dar.12473.

165. PhysicianGuideToBreadfeeding.org. Summary of ACR appropriateness criteria for breast imaging of pregnant and lactating women https:// eadn-wc01-5994650.nxedge.io/wp-content/uploads/2021/08 /ACRRecommendations.pdf

166. Ndikom CM, Fawole B, Ilesanmi RE. Extra fluids for breastfeeding mothers for increasing milk production. Cochrane Database Syst Rev. 2014;6(6):CD008758.

167. Palacios AM, Cardel MI, Parker E, Dickinson S, Houin VR, Young B, Allison DB. Effectiveness of lactation cookies on human milk production

rates: a randomized controlled trial. Am J Clin Nutr. 2023 May;117(5):1035–1042. doi: 10.1016/j.ajcnut.2023.03.010.

168. Foong SC, Tan ML, Foong WC, Marasco LA, Ho JJ, Ong JH. Oral galactagogues (natural therapies or drugs) for increasing breast milk production in mothers of non-hospitalised term infants. Cochrane Database Syst Rev. 2020 May 18;5(5):CD011505. doi: 10.1002/14651858 .CD011505.pub2.

169. https://www.breastfeedingnetwork.org.uk/factsheet/increasing-milk-supply -use-of-galactagogues/

170. Foong SC, Tan ML, Foong WC, Marasco LA, Ho JJ, Ong JH. Oral galactagogues (natural therapies or drugs) for increasing breast milk production in mothers of non-hospitalised term infants. Cochrane Database Syst Rev. 2020 May 18;5(5):CD011505. doi: 10.1002/14651858. CD011505.pub2.

171. Mitchell KB, Johnson HM, Rodríguez JM, Eglash A, Scherzinger C, Zakarija-Grkovic I, Cash KW, Berens P, Miller B; Academy of Breastfeeding Medicine. Academy of Breastfeeding Medicine Clinical Protocol #36: The Mastitis Spectrum, Revised 2022. Breastfeed Med. 2022 May;17(5):360–376. doi: 10.1089/bfm.2022.29207.kbm. Erratum in: Breastfeed Med. 2022 Nov;17(11):977–978.

172. Ibid.

173. Health and Safety Executive. Pregnant workers and new mothers: your health and safety https://www.hse.gov.uk/mothers/worker/index.htm

174. NHS. Types of formula, 2023 https://www.nhs.uk/conditions/baby /breastfeeding-and-bottle-feeding/bottle-feeding/types-of-formula/

175. NHS. Types of formula, 2023 https://www.nhs.uk/conditions/baby /breastfeeding-and-bottle-feeding/bottle-feeding/types-of-formula/

176. NHS. How to make up baby formula, 2022 https://www.nhs.uk /conditions/baby/breastfeeding-and-bottle-feeding/bottle-feeding/making -up-baby-formula/

177. NHS. Formula milk: common questions, 2019 https://www.nhs.uk /conditions/baby/breastfeeding-and-bottle-feeding/bottle-feeding/formula -milk-questions

178. InformedHealth.org. Cologne, Germany: Institute for Quality and Efficiency in Health Care (IQWiG); 2006. What is 'normal' sleep? 2013 [Updated 2016].

179. Grigg-Damberger MM. The visual scoring of sleep in infants 0 to 2 months of age. J Clin Sleep Med. 2016 Mar;12(3):429–445. doi: 10.5664 /jcsm.5600.

180. Grigg-Damberger MM, Wolfe KM. Infants sleep for brain. J Clin Sleep Med. 2017 Nov 15;13(11):1233–1234. doi: 10.5664/jcsm.6786.

181. Duncan JR, Byard RW. Sudden Infant Death Syndrome: an overview. In: Duncan JR, Byard RW, editors. SIDS sudden infant and early childhood death: the past, the present and the future. Adelaide (AU): University of Adelaide Press; 2018 May. Chapter 2.

182. Hauck FR, Thompson JM, Tanabe KO, Moon RY, Vennemann MM. Breastfeeding and reduced risk of Sudden Infant Death Syndrome: a meta-analysis. Pediatrics. 2011 Jul;128(1):103–110. doi: 10.1542/peds .2010-3000.

183. Alm B, Wennergren G, Möllborg P, Lagercrantz H. Breastfeeding and dummy use have a protective effect on Sudden Infant Death Syndrome. Acta Paediatr. 2016 Jan;105(1):31–38. doi: 10.1111/apa.13124.

184. National child Mortality Database. Sudden and unexpected deaths in infancy and childhood, 2022 https://www.ncmd.info/wp-content /uploads/2022/12/SUDIC-Thematic-report_FINAL.pdf

185. The Lullaby Trust. New survey shows 9 in 10 parents co-sleep but less than half know how to reduce the risk of SIDS, 2023 https://www.lullabytrust .org.uk/9-in-10-parents-co-sleep-but-less-than-half-know-how-to-reduce -the-risk-of-sids/

186. Middlemiss W, Granger DA, Goldberg WA, Nathans L. Asynchrony of mother–infant hypothalamic-pituitary-adrenal axis activity following extinction of infant crying responses induced during the transition to sleep. Early Hum Dev. 2012 Apr;88(4):227–232. doi: 10.1016/j.earlhumdev.2011.08.010.

187. Sadler S. Sleep: what is normal at six months? Prof Care Mother Child. 1994 Aug–Sep;4(6):166–167.

188. Pennestri MH, Burdayron R, Kenny S, Béliveau MJ, Dubois-Comtois K. Sleeping through the night or through the nights? Sleep Med. 2020 Dec;76:98–103. doi: 10.1016/j.sleep.2020.10.005.

189. Galland BC, Sayers RM, Cameron SL, Gray AR, Heath AM, Lawrence JA, Newlands A, Taylor BJ, Taylor RW. Anticipatory guidance to prevent infant sleep problems within a randomised controlled trial: infant, maternal and partner outcomes at 6 months of age. BMJ Open. 2017 Jun 2;7(5):e014908. doi: 10.1136/bmjopen-2016-014908.

190. Du Toit G, Roberts G, Sayre PH, Bahnson HT, Radulovic S, Santos AF, et al. Randomized trial of peanut consumption in infants at risk for peanut allergy. N Engl J Med. 2015;372(9):803–813.

191. Kuo AA, Inkelas M, Slusser WM, Maidenberg M, Halfon N. Introduction of solid food to young infants. Matern Child Health J. 2011 Nov;15(8): 1185–1194. doi: 10.1007/s10995-010-0669-5.

192. Section on Breastfeeding. Breastfeeding and the use of human milk. Pediatrics. 2012 Mar;129(3):e827–e841. doi: 10.1542/peds.2011-3552.

193. Grimshaw KE, Bryant T, Oliver EM, Martin J, Maskell J, Kemp T, Clare Mills EN, Foote KD, Margetts BM, Beyer K, Roberts G. Incidence and risk factors for food hypersensitivity in UK infants: results from a birth cohort study. Clin Transl Allergy. 2016 Jan 26;6:1. doi: 10.1186/s13601 -016-0089-8.

194. Sambrook J. Incidence of cow's milk protein allergy. Br J Gen Pract. 2016 Oct;66(651):512. doi: 10.3399/bjgp16X687277.

195. Du Toit G, Roberts G, Sayre PH, Bahnson HT, Radulovic S, Santos AF, et al. Randomized trial of peanut consumption in infants at risk for peanut allergy. N Engl J Med. 2015;372(9):803–813.

196. Perkin MR, Logan K, Marrs T, Radulovic S, Craven J, Flohr C, Lack G; EAT Study Team. Enquiring About Tolerance (EAT) study: feasibility of an early allergenic food introduction regimen. J Allergy Clin Immunol. 2016 May;137(5):1477–1486.e8. doi: 10.1016/j.jaci.2015.12.1322.

197. Gov.uk, Office for Health Improvement and Disparities. Summary of draft report: feeding young children aged 1 to 5 years, 2023 https://www.gov .uk/government/consultations/feeding-young-children-aged-1-to-5-years -draft-sacn-report/summary-of-draft-report-feeding-young-children-aged -1-to-5-years

198. NHS. NHS vaccinations and when to have them, 2023 https://www.nhs .uk/conditions/vaccinations/nhs-vaccinations-and-when-to-have-them/

199. NHS. MenB vaccine side effects, 2021 https://www.nhs.uk/conditions /vaccinations/men-b-vaccine-side-effects/

200. DeStefano F, Shimabukuro TT. The MMR vaccine and autism. Annu Rev Virol. 2019 Sep 29;6(1):585–600. doi: 10.1146/annurev-virology -092818-015515.

201. Shah V, Taddio A, McMurtry CM, Halperin SA, Noel M, Pillai Riddell R, Chambers CT; HELPinKIDS Team. Pharmacological and combined interventions to reduce vaccine injection pain in children and adults: systematic review and meta-analysis. Clin J Pain. 2015 Oct;31(10 Suppl): S38–S63. doi: 10.1097/AJP.0000000000000281.

202. Harrison D, Reszel J, Bueno M, Sampson M, Shah VS, Taddio A, Larocque C, Turner L. Breastfeeding for procedural pain in infants beyond the neonatal period. Cochrane Database Syst Rev. 2016 Oct 28;10(10): CD011248. doi: 10.1002/14651858.CD011248.pub2.

ACKNOWLEDGEMENTS

I would like to express my deepest gratitude to my husband, Rupert, whose unwavering support and understanding made it possible for me to delve into the world of 'author'. I know you must wish that I would just chill occasionally, but I love you for accepting that is just not my vibe. Your role as the father to our two wonderful children has not only enriched this book but also enriched my life.

To my mother, thank you for instilling in me the confidence to embark on the journey of motherhood. Your wisdom and love have been my guiding light, shaping not just this book but my entire approach to parenthood.

To my father, who has been the rock of our family. Your strength and compassion, especially during mum's illness, have been a source of inspiration. Your ability to nurture and care shines through not only in your role as a partner but also as a father and grandparent. Thank you for always being there, ready to answer any questions, provide guidance and share your knowledge. Your presence in my life has been a grounding force, and your resilience echoes in the pages of this book. This work is dedicated to you, Mum and Dad, as a tribute to the enduring bonds that shape our lives and the invaluable lessons on love, care and support that you've bestowed upon our family.

A heartfelt thank you to my dedicated agent, Alice, for championing this project and bringing it to fruition. Your expertise and enthusiasm have been invaluable.

I extend my appreciation to the incredible team at HarperCollins, especially Lydia, whose professionalism and passion have turned my ramblings into a tangible resource for expectant parents. Your commitment to excellence has truly brought *How to Have a Baby* to life.

Finally, to all my friends and family, and colleagues at 90 Sloane Street, who offered support, understanding, a listening ear and a cup of tea throughout this writing journey. Thank you for being my pillars of strength. I promise to see more of all of you now and stop using this book as an excuse for my non-attendance at gatherings.

This book is a testament to the collective efforts of those who believe in the transformative power of knowledge and the beauty of bringing new life into the world.

INDEX

A

abdominal pain 22, 57, 58, 114, 118
acid reflux 37, 39, 45, 233
active phase 102, 103, 122, 125
acupressure 24
acupuncture 9, 95, 115
adrenaline 103, 105, 120
advice, managing unsolicited 172–5
age 51
Akabusi, Shakira 35
alcohol: and breastfeeding 189, 199–202,
    212, 227
  in pregnancy 10–12, 13
  SIDS and 236, 237, 238, 239
allergies 252, 257, 261–4, 267, 276
alveoli 183, 226
amino acids 150
amniocentesis 51–2
amniotic fluid 44, 53, 101, 115
amniotic sac 43, 98, 99, 101
anaemia 17, 154
anaphylaxis 261, 276
angel kisses 141
animals 31
anomaly scans 47–50, 58
antenatal classes 68–70, 86, 175, 190–1
antenatal screening tests 50–2
anti-D immunoglobulin 18–19, 28
antibiotics 110, 111, 117, 132, 217
antibodies 73, 100, 186, 198
anal tears 111, 112, 135
anxiety: during labour 70, 72, 121, 122, 123
  and milk production 213
  postnatal 154
  in pregnancy 20, 34, 37
APGAR score 128, 179
areola 19, 74, 164, 183, 205
aromatherapy 121–2, 127
asphyxia, perinatal 119, 126
assisted delivery 110–13, 126

B

babies: breastfeeding 182–220, 227
  burping 195–7
  co-sleeping 201
  crying 195, 225
  effects of alcohol on 199–201
  feeding 182–228
  growth spurts 214
  hospital 'grab' bag 83–4
  low birth weight 52, 57
  milestones 280–6
  shoulder dystocia 119–20, 126
  sleep 229–50
  teething 268–73
  tongue-tie 189, 205, 206
  vaccinations 274–9
  weaning 198, 251–67
  see also foetus; newborn babies
baby blues 154–5, 180
baby-led weaning (BLW) 255–6, 257–8, 267
back to back position 111, 114
backs: back pain 33, 35, 45, 118
  exercising on your back 34
  sleeping on your 38, 39
balloon induction 98–100
bedtime routines 242, 250
bilirubin 112, 151
birth: position for 65, 126
  traumatic births 156–7
  where to give birth 65, 66–8
  see also labour
birth defects 8–9, 34
birth partners 65, 72
birth plans 64–6, 86, 89, 97
birth weight, low 12, 13, 52
birthing centres 67, 111, 144
birthing pools 67, 68, 88
birthmarks 139–41
bleeding: bleeding gums 27
  causes of in early pregnancy 57–8
  causes of in later pregnancy 58–9
  chorionic haemorrhage 58
  excessive bleeding 107
  following assisted delivery 111
  following External Cephalic Version (ECV) 114
  haemorrhagic disease of the newborn 131–2
  placental abruption 118
  postpartum 7, 105, 116–17, 126, 147, 187
  reduced bleeding 130
  unexpected bleeding 57–9, 63
  what to do if you are bleeding 59
blisters, milk 206
block feeding 214

blocked nose 27, 36
Blood Alcohol Concentration (BAC) 199–200
blood clots 7, 153
   chorionic haemorrhage 58
   deep vein thrombosis (DVT) 55, 56, 63, 107, 142
   following assisted delivery 111
   postpartum bleeding 147
   vitamin K 66
blood groups 17, 18
blood pressure 20, 105, 124
   high blood pressure 6, 17, 33, 55–6, 63, 73, 95
blood sampling, foetal 119
blood spot test 149–51, 180
blood sugar levels: baby's 73
   in early pregnancy 20, 23
   glucose tolerance test (GTT) 53–4
blood tests 17, 28, 50–1
Body Mass Index (BMI) 6, 7, 17
bonding 130–1
   see also skin-to-skin contact
booking visit 16–19, 28
bottle feeding 66, 168–9, 220–8
   choosing bottles and teats 222–3
   formula milk 191, 220–1, 251
   how much milk to give 224–5
   paced feeding 226, 227
   preparing formula feeds safely 221–2
   sterilising and cleaning bottles 223–4
   when to introduce 211
bowel movements: meconium 56, 73, 115, 126, 146
   postpartum 113, 136
   in labour 87–8, 101, 104
brain: development of 43, 45, 130, 150, 230
   perinatal asphyxia 119
breast milk 207, 251, 266
   alcohol in 199, 200–1
   boosting your supply 210–13, 228
   caffeine in 202
   colostrum harvesting 72–5
   composition of 184–5, 197–8, 226–7
   expressing 200–1, 217, 218
   insufficient supply 209–13, 228
   leaking 213
   milk supply 189, 201–2, 209–14, 228
   oversupply of 213–14, 228
   storage 202–4
   thawing frozen 203
breastfeeding 66, 73, 144, 182–220, 226–7
   alcohol and 199–202, 212, 227
   benefits of 185–7, 227
   block feeding 214
   breastfeeding to sleep 241, 244, 246, 247–8
   burping 195–7
   caffeine and 202, 227
   cluster feeding 187, 211, 214–15, 228
   co-sleeping and 239
   colostrum 72–5, 137
   composition of breast milk 184–5, 197–8, 226–7
   downsides of 187–9
   drop-off rates 198–9

establishing a strong breastfeeding relationship 192–7
evolution of the breastfeeding journey 197–9
exercise and 171–2
expressing 187–8, 207, 211
extended 188–9, 198
the first feed 136–7, 192
and hydration 179, 212
incessant feeding 214–15, 228
lactational amenorrhoea (LAM) 160, 161, 168
latching on 193, 205, 208–9, 211, 215, 227
low milk supply 209–13, 228
and low sex drive 159
mantras 189–90
milk supply 172, 209–14, 228
oversupply of breast milk 213–14, 228
physiological management of placenta 105
physiology of 183–4
positions for 193–4, 213
and postpartum bleeding 147
preparing for 190–2
in public 188–9, 218–19, 228
recognising hunger cues 194–5, 209
return of periods 168–9
returning to work 217–18, 228
SIDs and 237
skin-to-skin contact and 130
sleep myths 246
sore breasts 215–17, 228
sore nipples 204–7, 227
troubleshooting 204–20, 227–8
vitamin supplementation 266
breasts 183
   blocked ducts 213
   breast pain 153
   development of 226
   early pregnancy 19, 43
   engorgement 189, 214, 215
   mastitis 189, 213, 214, 215–16, 228
   milk leakage 45, 213
   postnatal changes 167, 181
   sore breasts 215–17, 228
   thrush 215
   see also nipples
breathing: breathing techniques 71, 121
   breathlessness 45
breech babies 106, 113, 114–15
burping your baby 195–7

C
Caesarean section (C-section) 106–8, 125
   delayed clamping 134
   elective 106–7
   emergency 7, 106, 107, 110–11, 112, 118, 119
   the first feed and 137
   induction and 97
   pain relief 142
   placenta praevia 59
   post 41-week pregnancies 96
   postpartum haemorrhage 117
   recovery from 108, 142–3, 154, 164, 180, 181
   risks of 107

what happens during 107–8
wound healing 108, 143, 154, 171
café-au-lait birthmarks 140
caffeine 21–2, 31–2, 189, 202, 227
candida 205–6
car seats 84, 145
cardiovascular health 21, 33
carriers 8–9, 13
catheters 111, 116, 124, 143
cervix: balloon induction 98–9
    bleeding in early pregnancy 58
    cervical sutures 73
    dilation of 95, 98, 101, 102, 103, 113, 123,
        125
    effacement 98, 99
    latent phase 101
    mucus plug 58, 101
    sweeps 98
cheese 30
choking 260, 264–5, 267
chorionic haemorrhage 58
chorionic villus sampling (CVS) 51–2
chromosomes 8–9, 43, 48
chronic disease 186, 187, 252
circadian rhythm 234, 245–6, 249
clothing: hospital wear 79, 80–1, 82, 143
    newborn baby's 83
cluster feeding 187, 211, 214–15, 228
co-sleeping 238–40
colostrum 72, 84, 130, 137, 183, 184, 227
    harvesting 72–5, 86
combined tests 51–2
complications in pregnancy 54–9
    deep vein thrombosis (DVT) 55, 56, 63
    Group B Streptococcus (GBS) 61–2, 63
    high blood pressure 55–6, 63
    hyperemesis gravidarum 56–7, 63
    intrahepatic cholestasis of pregnancy (ICP)
        56, 63
    reduced movements 44, 60
    unexpected bleeding 57–9, 63
conception 4–5, 9, 84
congenital abnormalities 31, 73, 138
congenital hypothyroidism 150
congenital moles 140
constipation 44, 113, 186
contact sports 34
contraception 9–10, 158–62, 180
contractions: active phase 102
    Braxton Hicks 45
    induced 99–100
    latent phase 101, 102, 125
    second stage of labour 103–4
    triggering 95
core muscles 33–4, 35, 36
cot death see Sudden Infant Death Syndrome
    (SIDS)
Covid-19 vaccinations 53
cow's milk 260, 261, 262
cow's milk protein allergy (CMPA) 262–3, 264
cramping 43, 44, 45, 57
cravings 26–7

crying: cry it out (CIO) method 240–1
    hunger cues 195, 225
    newborn babies 152
    tiredness 232
cystic fibrosis 8, 150

D
dates, inducing labour by eating 94
deep vein thrombosis (DVT) 55, 56, 63, 107,
    142
dehydration 25, 26, 56, 172
delivery, assisted 110–13, 126
dental care 27, 270–3
depression, postnatal (PND) 154–8, 159, 180
diabetes 6, 54, 95, 186, 187
    gestational 7, 17, 32, 33, 53–4, 56, 73
    perinatal asphyxia 119
diagnostic tests 48, 51–2, 119
diamorphine 123–4, 127
diarrhoea 186, 192, 262
diastasis recti 165, 181
diet 20–1, 25, 29–32, 94, 179
digestive system 186, 233
Down's syndrome 46, 51, 52
doxylamine 23, 24, 25
drooling 269, 270
due dates 62, 84–5, 86
dummies 211, 237
dysplasia, hip 138
dystocia, shoulder 119–20, 126

E
early pregnancy 16–28, 36, 43
eggs, fertilisation 43, 57
eggs (chicken's) 31, 259, 261, 262
electronic foetal monitoring (EFM) 118–19
embryos 43, 57–8
emotions 173, 178, 186–7
endorphins 21, 99–100, 122
engorgement 214, 215
Entonox 120, 123, 127
epidurals 100, 104, 108, 123, 124, 127, 135
episiotomy 65–6, 75, 104, 111, 112–13, 120,
    126, 134–6, 179
essential oils 121–2, 127
estimated due date (EDD) 84–5, 86
exercise: postnatal 170–2, 181
    in pregnancy 21, 33–6
expressing milk 187–8, 200–1, 207, 211, 217, 218
External Cephalic Version (ECV) 114
eyes 43, 44, 138

F
family 40–1, 174, 172–7
    family history 8–9, 13
fatigue 20–2, 36, 43, 159, 233
feeding your baby 66, 182–228
    breastfeeding 182–220, 226–7
    formula feeding 220–8
fertilisation 57, 84
fertility 9–10, 11, 12, 158
fingernails, development of 43, 44

first trimester 20, 23, 32, 34
  causes of bleeding in 57–8
  growth of foetus 43–4
  increased urinary frequency 22, 43
  tests and scans 46–7, 50–2
fish 30, 189, 192, 261
flu vaccinations 52
foetal alcohol syndrome (FAS) 12, 13
foetus: abnormal heart rate 118–19, 126
  effect of alcohol on 12, 13
  effect of caffeine on 22
  first trimester 43–4
  foetal blood sampling 119
  foetal distress 107, 115
  growth of 41–5
  meconium 56, 115, 126
  movement of 44, 60
  perinatal asphyxia 119, 126
  position of 114–15, 126
  risk of stillbirth 38
  second trimester 44–5
  size of 42
  third trimester 45
  weight of 44–5
folic acid 5–6, 12, 13, 37, 43, 164
foods: forbidden foods in pregnancy 29–32
  ready-prepared baby food 260–1
  spicy food 94
  teething relief 270
  weaning 251–67
forceps 110, 111, 113
foremilk 185
formula feeding 191, 220–8, 251
fourth trimester 130, 152–3
friends 40–1, 172–7
full-term pregnancy 84, 86, 95, 96
fundus 196–7

G
gagging 264–5, 267
galactagogues 212–13
gas and air 120, 123, 127
gastro-esophageal reflux disease (GORD) 233
gender, identifying 47, 48–50
genes, broken 8–9, 13
genitalia 47, 139
gestational diabetes mellitus (GDM) 7, 32, 33,
  53–4, 56, 73
gestational hypertension 55–6, 154
ginger 23–4
glucose tolerance test (GTT) 53–4
glutaric aciduria type 1 (GA1) 150–1
GPs 14, 149, 153–4, 158, 171, 180
Group B Streptococcus (GBS) 61–2
growth, fetal 12, 13, 142
gums 27, 270

H
haemangiomas 141
haemorrhage: chorionic haemorrhage 58
  postpartum haemorrhage (PPH) 105, 116–17,
    126, 147

haemorrhagic disease of the newborn 131–2
hair: lanugo 44, 45
  postnatal changes 167, 181
hearing screen 137–8
heart (baby's) 48, 138
  heart rate 45, 97, 114, 118–19, 126
heartburn 45, 94
heel prick test 149–51, 180
hepatitis B 17, 28, 50–1, 208
hindmilk 185
hips: NIPE screening 138
  postnatal 163, 180–1
HIV 17, 28, 50, 208
home births 68, 87–93, 144, 145
homocystinuria (pyridoxine unresponsive)
  (HCU) 151
honey 259
hormones 11, 36, 44, 58, 159, 230
  in early pregnancy 19, 20, 27, 36
  see also individual hormones
hospital 'grab' bag 79–84
hospitals: choosing 14–16, 28
  discharge from 143–5
  labour ward 67
  neonatal units 144–5
Huichol people 66
hunger cues, recognising 194–5, 209, 225
hydration 25, 26, 179, 212
hyperemesis gravidarum 23, 56–7, 63
hypertension, gestational 55–6, 154
hypnobirthing 66, 70–2, 86, 120
hypothyroidism, congenital 150

I
ibuprofen 9, 135, 216–17
immune system (baby's) 45, 73, 186, 198, 274
immune system (mother's) 52–3
implantation 43, 57–8, 84
incontinence, urinary 77, 111
induction 85, 86, 94–100
infections 58, 111, 117, 136
  benefits of breastfeeding 186, 252
  neonatal 109, 110, 151
inferior vena cava (IVC) 39, 166
intrahepatic cholestasis of pregnancy (ICP) 56,
  63, 95
iron 21, 37, 133, 233, 251, 258
isovaleric acidaemia (IVA) 150

J
jaundice 53, 56, 73, 111–12, 133, 134, 149,
  151–2, 180
juice 260

L
labour 87–127
  abnormal heart rate of the baby 118–19,
    126
  active phase 102, 122, 125
  assisted delivery 110–13, 126
  baby's position 114–15, 126
  birthing positions 125

bringing on naturally 86
complications of 125–6
episiotomy 65–6, 75, 104, 111, 112–13, 120, 126, 134–6, 179
first stage of labour 101–3, 125
hypnobirthing 70–2, 86
induced 85, 86, 95–100
latent phase 122, 125
meconium 115, 126
monitoring during 65, 99
perinatal asphyxia 119, 126
perineal tears 75, 90, 104, 111, 112, 113, 116, 117, 126, 134–6, 179
placental abruption 118, 126
postpartum haemorrhage (PPH) 116–17, 126
precipitous labour 116, 126
premature rupture of membranes (PROM) 109–10, 125
pushing stage 89, 103, 104, 110, 125
retained placenta 117, 126
second stage of labour 103–4, 124, 125
shoulder dystocia 119–20, 126
signs of early labour 87–8
slow progression 113, 126
stages of 100–6, 125
third stage of labour 105–6, 122, 125
transition phase 103, 122, 125
troubleshooting 108–20
what brings labour on 94–5
see also Caesarean section; pain relief
labour preparation 33–4, 64–86
birth plans 64–6, 86, 89
colostrum harvesting 72–5, 86
due dates 84–5, 86
hospital 'grab' bag 79–84
pelvic floor exercises 76–9, 86
perineal massage 75–6, 86
where to give birth 65, 66–8
labour ward 67, 111, 144
lanolin 83, 206–7
lanugo 44, 45
latent phase 101–2, 122, 125
legs, Restless Leg Syndrome (RLS) 37
libido 44, 159
ligaments 35, 171
linea nigra 136, 164
listeria 30, 31
liver 39, 56, 199
Local Neonatal Unit (LNU) 144
lochia 147, 171, 210
lungs 44, 45, 100, 139

M
maple syrup urine disease (MSUD) 150
massage 72, 121
perineal massage 75–6, 112
mastitis 189, 213, 214, 215–16, 228
mature milk 184–5, 227
meats to avoid 30–1
meconium 56, 73, 115, 126, 146
medication 9–10, 13, 24–5, 123–4, 156

medium-chain acyl-CoA dehydrogenase deficiency (MCADD) 150
membranes, amniotic 98
rupture of 73, 99, 101, 109–10, 113, 125
MenB vaccine 275, 276
menstrual cycles 5, 7, 9–10
postnatal 168–70, 181
mental health 16, 154–8, 159, 180
midwifes 16–19, 28, 149
milestones 280–6
milk blisters 206
milk ducts 183, 215, 226
mindfulness 156
miscarriage 7, 30, 31–2, 58
definition of 57
percentage of pregnancy ending in 40
reasons for 41
risk of diagnostic tests 51–2
MMR vaccine 275, 276–7
moles, congenital 140
Mongolian blue spots 140
morning sickness 22–6, 43
hyperemesis gravidarum 23, 56–7, 63
mortality 97, 107
see also miscarriage; stillbirths
mothers: breastfeeding 182–220, 227
hospital 'grab' bag 79–83
the postnatal body 162–7, 180–1
postnatal exercise 170–2, 181
postnatal periods 168–70, 181
pre-pregnancy 4–13
pregnancy 14–63
self-care 177–9
sex and contraception 158–62, 180, 187
support networks 172–7
movement: during labour 123, 127
foetal movements 44, 60
NIPE screening 139
moxibustion 114–15
muscles: core muscles 33–4, 35, 36
diastasis recti 165, 181
NIPE screening 139

N
Naevus of Ota birthmarks 140
nappies 148, 210
nausea see morning sickness
Neonatal Intensive Care Unit (NICU) 144–5
neonatal sepsis 61, 192
neural tube 5–6, 13, 43
newborn babies: 6–8-week postnatal check 153–4, 158, 180
APGAR score 128–9, 179
birthmarks 139–41
blood spot test 149–51, 180
bottle feeding 223, 224
clamping and cutting the cord 106, 108, 125, 132–4, 179
cord care 151, 180
crying 152
first 24 hours 145–7
the first feed 136–7, 146, 183, 192

newborn babies (*continued*)
full newborn health check 138–9, 180
hearing screen 137–8
immune systems 274, 279
jaundice 53, 73, 111–12, 133, 134, 149,
151–2, 180
meconium and poo 73, 115, 126, 146
nappies 146, 148
recognising hunger cues 195, 209, 225
skin-to-skin contact 108, 129–31, 136, 179,
192, 209
sleep 145–6, 178, 230–2, 234, 249
vitamin K 131–2, 179
Newborn and Infant Physical Examination
(NIPE) 138–9, 180
nipples 19, 136, 153, 183, 210
nipple stimulation 95
sore nipples 189, 204–7, 208, 227
non-invasive prenatal testing (NIPT) 51
nuchal translucency (NT) 46, 51, 52
nuts 260, 261

O
occiput-posterior position 111, 114
oestrogen 7, 37, 98, 159, 164, 167
and milk production 19, 183, 226
ovulation 4–5, 7, 9, 11, 168
oxytocin 105, 116, 130
breastfeeding 183, 187
labour 94, 95, 98, 99, 120
placental delivery 90, 105
synthetic 99, 105, 113, 125

P
paced feeding 226, 227
pain: abdominal pain 22, 57, 58, 114, 118
active management of placenta 105
and sleep disturbances 233
pain relief: assisted deliveries 111
C-sections 142
episiotomy 113
hypnobirthing 70–2
inductions and 99–100
in labour 65, 67, 68, 120–4, 126–7
managing perineal tears 135
medication 123–4
relaxation 121–3
teething 270
paracetamol 135, 216–17
parent-led weaning (PLW) 255–6, 267
peanuts 252, 261, 264
pelvic floor 36, 77
exercises 76–9, 86, 154, 171
pelvis, postnatal 35–6, 163
peri-bottles 82, 135–6
perinatal asphyxia 119, 126
perineum: episiotomy 65–6, 75, 104, 111,
112–13, 120, 126
perineal healing 154
perineal massage 75–6, 86, 112
perineal tears 75, 90, 104, 111, 112, 113, 116,
117, 126, 134–6, 179

periods, postnatal 168–70, 181
pethidine 123–4, 127
phenylketonuria (PKU) 150
phototherapy 134, 151
pigmented birthmarks 140
pineapple 95
placenta 20, 22, 98, 132, 183
chorionic haemorrhage 58
chorionic villus sampling (CVS) 51
cord clamping 106, 133
delivery of 66, 90, 105, 106, 108, 116
development of 43, 44
physiological management 105, 106, 117
placenta praevia 58, 59, 106, 117, 119
placental abruption 59, 117, 118, 119, 126
position of 46, 58, 59
retained placenta 116, 117, 126
third stage of labour 105, 125, 130, 183
pneumonia 52, 61, 192
port wine stains 141
postnatal 128–81
postnatal depression (PND) 154–8, 159, 180
postnatal wards 144
postpartum haemorrhage (PPH) 105, 116–17,
126, 147, 187
postpartum psychosis 157–8
pre-eclampsia 7, 17, 32, 53, 55–6, 106, 117, 119,
154
pre-pregnancy 4–13
precipitous labour 116, 126
preconception 5–13
pregnancy 14–63
anomaly scan 47–50, 58, 62–3
antenatal screening tests 50–2
baby's growth 41–5
complications in 54–62, 63
due dates 43, 84–5, 86
early pregnancy 14–28, 43–4
exercise in 33–6, 62
first trimester 3–4
forbidden foods 29–32, 62
glucose tolerance test (GTT) 53–4, 63
Group B Streptococcus (GBS) 61–2, 63
reduced foetal movements 60
second trimester 44–5
sleep in 36–9, 62
telling friends and family 40–1
third trimester 45
12–week scan 46–7, 62–3
vaccinations 52–3, 63
weight in 32–3, 62
premature birth 7, 12, 13, 32, 52, 53, 58, 85,
118
premature rupture of membranes (PROM)
109–10, 125
preterm premature ruptured membranes
(PPROM) 73, 109, 110
progesterone 20, 22, 98, 159, 164
effect on sleep 36, 37
and milk production 19, 183, 226
prolactin 19, 159, 183–4, 226
prostaglandin 87–8, 94, 98, 99, 170

psychosis, postpartum 157–8
pulmonary embolism (PE) 55
pushing stage 89, 103, 104, 110, 125

Q
quadruple blood screening 52

R
raspberry leaf tea 94
red blood cells 18–19, 28, 50
the Red Book 141–2, 276
reflexes 100, 138, 139, 253
   development of 44, 45
   gagging reflex 265
reflux 37, 39, 45, 233
relaxation 35, 70–2, 121–3, 126, 156
relaxin 23, 35, 163, 171
Remifentanil 124, 127
resistance training 33–4, 35
respiratory distress 115
Restless Leg Syndrome (RLS) 37
rhesus disease 18–19, 28
rhinitis, pregnancy 27, 36
ribs, postnatal 163, 180–1
rice cereal 245–6
rooting reflex 195
routines, bedtime 242, 250
Rusty Pipe Syndrome 208

S
salmon patches 141
salmonella 31
salt 259
scans: anomaly scans 47–50, 58
   gender identification 44
   nuchal translucency scan 46
   12–week scan 46–7
   ultrasound 17
screening tests: anomaly scan 47–50, 58
   antenatal screening tests 50–2
   blood tests 50–1
   combined tests 51–2
   full newborn health check 138–9, 180
   hearing screen 137–8
   non-invasive prenatal testing (NIPT) 51
   quadruple blood screening 52
   12–week scan 46–7
second trimester 20, 32, 44–5, 52, 53
self-care 177–9
self-soothing 240–1
sepsis 61, 192
sex: during pregnancy 58, 94
   postnatal 158–62, 180
shellfish 30, 259
shoulder dystocia 119–20, 126
shows 58, 101
sickle cell disease 8, 50, 149
6–8-week postnatal check 153–4, 158, 171, 180
skin, postnatal changes 45, 164–6, 181
skin-to-skin contact 65, 108, 129–31, 136, 179, 192, 209
   breastfeeding and 186

following assisted delivery 112
   physiological management of placenta 105
sleep: babies and 229–50
   bedtime routines 242, 250
   breastfeeding to sleep 241, 244, 246, 247–8
   co-sleeping 201, 238–40
   coping with sleep challenges 240–8
   creating sleep-inviting environments 243, 250
   cry it out (CIO) method 240–1
   during pregnancy 20, 21, 34, 36–9
   excessive daytime sleepiness 232
   importance of sleep 229–30, 249
   newborn babies 178, 249
   postnatal 178
   red flags 232–3, 244, 249
   rice cereal myth 245–6
   seeking help 244, 250
   sleep cues 243, 250
   sleep cycles 230–2, 249
   sleep myths 245–8
   sleep progression 233–5, 249–50
   sleeping positions 37, 38–9
   sleeping through the night (STTN) 245, 247
   Sudden Infant Death Syndrome (SIDS) 235–7, 238, 239–40, 250
   trying out new timings 243, 250
sleep apnoea 36, 233
smoking 236, 237, 238, 239
snoring 36, 39, 232
Special Care Baby Unit (SCBU) 144
spicy food 94
spine 43, 139
spotting, implantation 43, 57–8
squats 33–4, 35
sterilising and cleaning bottles 223–4
stillbirth 7, 30, 38, 39, 53, 56, 96, 118
stitches 108, 113, 134–5
stomach acid 23, 37, 39, 45, 233
stork bites 141
strawberry marks 141
stress 11, 130, 213
stretch marks 45, 165–6
sucking reflex 45
Sudden Infant Death Syndrome (SIDS) 97, 201, 235–7, 238, 239–40, 250
sugar 259
support networks 174, 175–7
swallowing reflex 44, 45, 100
sweeps 98
swimming 34, 171
syphilis 17, 28, 50, 51

T
tea 32
tears: anal 112, 135
   perineal 75, 90, 111, 112, 113, 116, 117, 126, 134–6, 179
   reducing risk of 104
teats 223
teeth: teething 268–73
   tooth care 27, 270–3
teething 268–73

TENS machines (Transcutaneous Electrical Nerve Stimulation) 120, 123, 127
testes 44, 45, 138
thalassaemia 50
therapy 156
thiamine 56
third trimester 20, 32, 45
thrush 58, 205–6, 215
thyroid gland 150
tongue thrust reflex 253
tongue-tie 189, 205, 206
toxoplasmosis 30–1
Traditional Chinese Medicine 24, 114–15
transition phase 103, 122, 125
transitional care 145
transitional milk 184, 227
traumatic births 156–7
tummy time 281
12-week scan 46–7
20-week scan see anomaly scan
twins 134
type 2 diabetes 54, 186, 187

U
ultra-processed foods 260
ultrasound scans 17, 46, 47–50, 58
umbilical cord: clamping 106, 108, 125, 132, 133–4, 179
  compression of 119
  cord care 133, 151, 180
  cutting the cord 65, 132–4, 179
  NIPE screening 139
  snapping of 117
urinary tract infections (UTIs) 22, 26
urination: catheters 111, 116, 124, 143
  epidurals and 124
  incontinence 77, 111
  increased frequency 22, 43
  newborn babies 146
  peri-bottles 82, 136

V
vaccinations 52–3, 142, 274–9
vacuum cups 110
vaginal births: following C-sections 107
  see also labour
varicose veins 166
vasa praevia 59
vascular birthmarks 140–1
vegetables 21, 260

veins: deep vein thrombosis (DVT) 55, 56, 63, 107, 142
  piles 45
  varicose veins 166
ventouse 110, 111, 113
vernix 44, 45, 129
visualisation techniques 70–2
vitamins 192, 266
  vitamin A 31, 184, 266
  vitamin B 5, 56
  vitamin B6 23–4, 25
  vitamin C 21, 258, 266
  vitamin D 192, 266
  vitamin K 66, 131–2, 179, 184
  vitamin K deficiency bleeding (VKDB) 131–2
vomiting see morning sickness

W
water births 122–3, 127
waters: breaking of 99, 101, 109, 113, 125
  premature membrane rupture (PROM) 109–10
  preterm premature ruptured membranes (PPROM) 73, 109, 110
weaning 198, 251–67
  allergies 261–4, 267
  baby-led weaning (BLW) 255–6, 257–8, 267
  choking versus gagging 264–5, 267
  foods to avoid 259–60, 267
  foods to start with 257–9
  parent-led weaning (PLW) 256, 267
  preparing for weaning 253–5
  ready-prepared baby food 260–1
  reasons for weaning 251–2
  sleep myths 245–6
  vitamin supplementation 266
  when to wean 252–3, 267
weight (baby's) 31–2, 53, 142, 210
weight (foetus's) 44–5
weight (mother's) 6–7, 13, 32–3, 56
weights, lifting heavy 35
whooping cough 52–3
work, returning to 217–18, 228

Y
yoga 34
'you' time 177

Z
zygotes 43